MW00877812

Redesign Your Life
A Blueprint For Health

Kathleen J. Stricker

Certified Traditional Naturopath

Certified Nutritional Consultant

VoiceBio™ Sound Therapist

REDESIGN YOUR LIFE: A BLUEPRINT FOR HEALTH

Copyright © 2016 by Kathleen J. Stricker. All rights reserved.

Cover photography by Autumn R. DiScala.

No part of this book may be reproduced or transmitted in any form or by any means, electronic or mechanical, including photocopying, recording, or by an information storage and retrieval system, without written permission from the publisher.

Product names, brands, and other trademarks referred to within this book are the property of their respective trademark holders. These trademark holders are not affiliated with and do not sponsor or endorse this book, its contents, or its author.

Printed in the United States of America.

ISBN: 152399133X

ISBN-13: 978-1523991334

FIRST EDITION, REVISED

www.daystarnatural.com

TABLE OF CONTENTS

All information is for educational purposes only and is not intended for diagnosis of disease. Do not attempt to diagnose yourself. Consult with a qualified professional for proper assessment of imbalances.

Introduction

Instead of relying on traditional broken healthcare systems, Americans are searching for alternative solutions to their health problems. Herbal remedies, dietary changes, vitamins, minerals, and exercise are some of the venues that attract those people. (April 20, 2012 – The Centers for Disease Control and Prevention confirms this search: "More of half of U.S. adults use dietary supplements – including multivitamins, minerals, and herbs.")

Although there are some who feel better and do make progress, the questions remain, "Am I wasting my money? Is there something missing?" Without education and proper training, health targets are misdirected, and goals are not achieved, resulting in frustration and confusion.

In spite of this determination to achieve good health naturally, the general population shows evidence of more degenerative diseases than ever before. On September 18, 2012, ABC News stated, "By 2030, more than half of Americans could be obese, resulting in millions of new cases of diabetes, coronary heart disease, and stroke."

Despite warnings from the Attorney General, cigarette smoking alone accounts for about 443,000 deaths (almost one of out of every five) each year in the U.S. and is independently responsible for approximately 20% of strokes and about 35% of all heart attacks, particularly fatal ones.

Fox news, January 15, 2013: "Cigarette smoking and obesity are proven to increase risk for serious diseases, worsen outcomes from those diseases, and decrease life expectancy – even with excellent medical care. And their impact is huge."

Because smoking harms nearly every organ of the body, it causes or exacerbates many additional diseases, and it worsens outcomes from surgery and innumerable other treatments.

Obesity is now linked to greater risk of death from heart disease, stroke, diabetes, high blood pressure, all of the most prevalent cancers, and worse treatment outcomes after heart surgery, trauma and burn surgery, and transplants. It is not simply that rates of diseases are higher; the treatment outcomes are significantly worse for cigarette smokers and obese patients."

We purposely neglect to investigate the damages of the Standard American Diet (SAD). We meet socially for business purposes, parties, celebrations, dating, or just to have a night out. Restaurants cook with processed ingredients, and in some cases, the food is so overcooked that there is no nutritional value left. It is "dead" food. In addition, the portions are much larger than our stomachs can hold. But considering the cost of the meal, we force ourselves to eat the larger serving anyway!

As children we were introduced to traditional and ethnic foods and especially overeat during the holidays. We eat meals while working, watching television, listening to the radio, or reading a book or newspaper. We gobble our food instead of taking time to chew each bite and enjoy, or even taste, our foods. Some people may eat during an emotional crisis as a way to soothe nerves. All of these reasons are why many Americans are overweight.

America has adopted the western model of medicine, which prescribes medications and embraces surgeries or other invasive techniques. Most medical doctors and trained professionals are caught between insurance regulations and a public that demands a quick fix in order to continue the abuse that harmed the body in the first place.

Most people make a change in diet and lifestyles only when they are faced with a chronic discomfort or a life-threatening illness or pain. Some people become dissatisfied with their condition and, with determination, find a trained health professional to coach them back to health.

The mission and aim of DayStar Natural, LLC is to help healthy individuals prevent disease and sickness and to restore health to those who have health challenges. We work as a team with our clients to help make those changes physically, psychologically, and spiritually through clinically supported nutritional programs.

Based on the principle that healing takes place from the inside out, DayStar Natural, LLC believes that only whole, living foods and quality nutritional support will repair the body. Because we care about families, we believe that we can provide affordable, quality healthcare without the use of surgery and drugs. We have helped thousands regain good health and stay healthy.

Introduction

CHAPTER 1

My Journey to Health

I was raised in western Pennsylvania where my Hungarian grandparents struggled to support their six children by farming. My father was tall, strong, and a hard worker. I was short, sickly, and felt fatigued most of my life.

I was prone to colds, flu symptoms, allergies, and digestive distress. My mother informed me that she had to wipe my infant eyes with a warm cloth each morning in order to clear the sticky, crusty mucus that accumulated around my eyes every night.

When I was 10 years old, my parents and my family doctor made the decision to remove my tonsils to alleviate earaches and sore throats. The procedure did not cure anything. I continued to experience laryngitis and bronchitis over the next several years, especially every fall season.

Although a healthy, normal bowel movement should occur no less than once a day (three times is optimum), I was often bloated, gassy, and constipated. My bowel movements occurred once a week and sometimes once every other week.

I had a weight problem as a teenager, which contributed to my insecurities. I craved carbohydrates and sugar, especially chocolate. I was only 5 feet tall and weighed 125 lbs plus, but I could eat as much as my father who was 6 feet tall and weighed 215 lbs. How embarrassing when I went to college and was "auctioned off" at an initiation event during freshman week as "The Battle of The Bulge."

While in college, I managed to hide my insecurities long enough to have a relationship and get married. After I had my first child at age 20, I had severe pains in my back. Standing for more than

15 minutes, caused a pinching, burning sensation that would radiate down my left leg from my hip joint to my knee. I would stretch my leg or lean against a wall to get temporary relief.

Mentally, I felt overwhelmed, confused, and foggy, and it was an effort to understand concepts. I would read an article and immediately forget what I had read. I could not repeat or duplicate anything. I felt like my brain was clogged. My head was spinning with ideas, but I could not translate those ideas into practical applications.

I lived with headaches for years. Even in elementary school I was given baby aspirin frequently due to these headaches. I would see silver stars in my "aura" and was light-headed and dizzy when bending over. Although I was never diagnosed, I believe these were migraine headaches.

I continued to take pain killers as an adult almost daily to ward off even a hint of a headache. Throbbing headaches would persist for two weeks to a month non-stop. Several times I would wake up in the middle of the night with stabbing, frightening, "icepick" headaches. These headaches would interfere with my life. I could not think clearly when my head was pounding, and I avoided doing certain activities, which would intensify the pain.

I was sneezing and wheezing every day all year long, regardless of the season. My nasal passages were constantly blocked, and I breathed out of my mouth the majority of the time. I tried various methods to unblock my sinuses such as using a face mask to steam the sinuses open or a hair dryer thinking it would dry them up. An allergy specialist concluded that I had several airborne allergies. So, for over 14 years, my arms were like pincushions with four injections a week (two in each arm) to desensitize the allergies. The procedure did not resolve my allergies. It seemed to make the symptoms worse!

Not only was breathing difficult, but so was sleep. I had restless legs, itchy skin, and itchy scalp. The frustration of looking at the clock all night long, tossing and turning from skin irritations and trouble- some, worrisome thoughts swirling around in my head made me one miserable person! The alarm would go off just as I would fall asleep, and the sleep deprivation caused me to be irritable.

 My eyes were sunken in, and my face was pale and pasty-looking. By noon my makeup had worn off, and I looked like death warmed over. My nerves were frazzled, I had acid indigestion, constipation, hemorrhoids, itchy eyes and ears, painful blisters in my mouth, and a lump in my throat from anxiety and stress. I thought I would be exhausted from a self-inflicted exercise - running up and down stairs several times - but that only created more stress and more insomnia since it seemed to rev me up even more!

For a period of approximately one year, both my thumbs were so swollen and inflamed (twice their normal size) that I could not bend them. I would find ways to compensate for the pain - trying various techniques and natural therapies.

At bed time I would rub essential oils into the joints and hold the vials gently to fall asleep. When the essential oils wore off, I would wake up with burning pain and numbness down my hands, wrists, and elbows. I shook my hands vigorously until the circulation came back.

I tried lymphatic patches to pull toxins out of my wrists and thumbs. Instead of placing the patches on the bottom of my feet first per the instructions, I affixed the patches to my wrists or thumbs. If there were no toxins, the patches would come off clean the next morning. If there was some junk, the patches were dark brown and gooey!

Once I woke up with such a throbbing pain in my thumb that I ripped the patches off, ran to the bathroom, and ran cold water over my thumb for an hour before it cooled down. It felt as if there was a red-hot copper rod in place of the bone. My husband suggested that I go to see a medical doctor. My reply, "Read my lips! No!" I was determined to find an answer myself.

I went regularly to a chiropractor, and in one of our conversations, we concluded that I was detoxing copper through my thumbs. I had been receiving allergy shots (2 in each arm every week) for over 14 years, which most likely had been made with a copper base.

I have had several surgeries: a tonsillectomy at age 10, a hysterectomy to remove a lemon-sized fibroid tumor at age 44, a partial mastectomy to remove a blocked duct, and a surgery to correct a deviated septum. I took over-the-counter antihistamines to breathe, acetaminophen and chiropractic care for pain, laxatives for constipation, vitamin C (ascorbic acid) for allergies, vitamin B for energy, calcium for osteopenia/osteoporosis, and antacids for indigestion. I was masking my symptoms, and nothing ever changed or improved. By 1994, I was frustrated, exhausted, worn out, and fatigued.

I was taught to respect and never question the education of traditional medical doctors and drug companies. Unfortunately, that thinking did not help my older brother who passed away from cancer at age 56. I witnessed his strong muscles vanish and his handsome features cave in as the chemotherapy ravaged his frame. When the doctor stood at his bedside and stated, "Well, Larry, you only have about a day and a half to live.", Larry responded in shock, "Doc, I thought you were going to fix me." Knowing that is the typical response of a drug dependent nation, I knew there had to be a better way.

In 1997, my husband and I were on a mission trip to New Mexico to conduct Junior Youth Camp for Navajo Indian children. During our visit, the team toured Canyon de Chelley National Park. The walk down the canyon was a mile long as we hugged the crooked, steep, rocky path. It was hot, and the sun was strong. I made the trip down with a little difficultly, but on the way back up, my husband literally had to pull me up the mountain.

One of our team members referred me to her nutritionist and shared how she had been helped with similar symptoms. I was not receptive to healing with nutrition at first, but I went out of desperation. That was my introduction to a holistic approach and alternative medicine.

The naturopath was suspicious that my immune challenges were related to parasites. He said I was a perfect host for parasites since I was very acidic. He recommended some herbs and whole food supplements, and I started on his program. Within weeks, I began seeing positive changes. That was the beginning of my healing without the use of toxic drugs and the side effects.

Once I was on a good nutritional program, I started to detox all the chemicals from years of over-the-counter medications. Although detoxing did not feel good at the time, once I cleared the toxins, my health started turning around, and I finally had some color in my cheeks. I never knew how sick I really was until I became healthy.

Other people saw changes in me and wanted to know if I could help them. I tried but soon learned that it was not one-size-fits-all, quick-fix remedies. Initially I started taking classes just to help myself and my family. The first course I enrolled in was in 1998. "Certified Herbal Consultant" was written by the founder of Tree of Life Publishing, Steven Horne, a member and past president of the American Herbalists Guild.

I began teaching and sharing my limited understanding of natural therapies with a small group of people in 1999. After a few months, one of the ladies in the class came to me excitedly reporting that her doctor declared her Crohn's disease was gone! He gave her a clean bill of health, and all I did was teach a few basic principles about health!

After two years into the training, I felt like I had to go into a new and unfamiliar area of research to reclaim my health and the health of others, just as David in 1 Samuel 30* had to take back all that had been stolen from him. This training was strange, but

---

*"Now the Amelekites had raided the Negev and Ziklag. They had attacked Ziklag and burned it, and had taken captive the women and all who were in it, both young and old. They killed none of them, but carried them off as they went on their way. When David and his men came to Ziklag, they found it destroyed by fire and their wives and sons and daughters taken captive. So David and his men wept aloud until they had no strength left to weep. David was greatly distressed because the men were talking of stoning him; each one was bitter in spirit because of his sons and daughters. But David found strength in the LORD his God." *I Samuel 30:1-6 NIV*

"David recovered everything the Amalekites had taken, including his two wives. Nothing was missing: young or old, boy or girl, plunder or anything else they had taken. David brought everything back." *I Samuel 30: 18-19 NIV*

there was a purpose for all the challenges that I faced, and I started moving to a level higher than I could ever imagine.

I continued to pursue learning about natural solutions and techniques even though I was not thoroughly convinced that herbs and vitamins worked. I had studied for four years before it became evident to me that the correct application of natural therapy is safe and effective.

From 2000 to 2002, I traveled the east coast pursuing hands-on training from Certified National Health Professionals (cnhp.org). These capstone classes included: Iridology, Sclerology, Parasitology, Aromatherapy, Flower Essence Therapy, Light Touch Therapy, Nutrition, Body Systems, Anatomy and Physiology, Muscle Testing, Face-Tongue-Nail Analysis, Homeopathy, Enzyme Therapy, and Survival Techniques.

In 2002, I was trained by Kae Thompson-Liu (VIBEprints™ Corporation, Roanoke, VA, voicebio.com) as a VoiceBio® Sound Therapist. In between studies, I studied and practiced Stress Management techniques taught by Bob Miller – Tree of Life Health Ministries, Denver, PA – into 2003.

Since 2004, I have traveled to Chicago, California, Philadelphia, Atlanta, Austin, and various other locations to study Quantum Reflex Analysis and Vastu Remediation (Dr. Robert Marshall, Dr. Linda Forbes of Premier Research Labs, Austin, Texas).

Other accreditation include Hydrocolon Therapy (Helen Wood Institute, Kissimmee, Florida, 2005); Theophostic Prayer Ministry (Dr. Ed Smith, Campbellsville, KY 2007); The Ki Method and the Physics and Science of BioElectrical Energy (Glenn King, Carrollton, Texas, 2008).

From 2003 to 2007, I studied to be a Certified Traditional Naturopath and Certified Nutritional Consultant from Trinity School of Natural Health (Warsaw, Indiana, www.trinityschool.org).

Although I helped a few people, it was not enough to justify the reason for becoming a health care practitioner. I was frustrated because my initial analysis and consultation usually lasted two hours or more. I was uncertain about the direct cause of the symptoms, so I tried to support every area of the body. The cost of supplements alone would cost approximately $250 to $750 for one visit. People rarely returned and I had no feedback to verify that my protocols were working.

It was during a class in May 2008 that I met a young lady who was using Nutrition Response Testing™ to evaluate other class members during our lunch break. Her approach addressed the source of pain and discomfort and supported solutions for healing. When I asked her about her approach, she stated, "Ah, you already know everything!" When I contradicted her and insisted she had the information that I needed, she pointed me to this technology that had been missing in my training.

In October 2008, I started taking courses from Ulan Nutritional Systems, which included both Basic and Intermediate Training. In 2009, I attended the first phase of the Advanced Clinical Training (ACT) from January to June under Dr. Ulan's colleague, Dr. Lester Bryman. I took the ACT refresher course from April to September 2010 and completed the training with the ACT booster course from January to May 2012. I received the Ulan "Wall of Fame" award in December 2012 for reaching his expectations and goals for graduates.

Before I learned about Nutrition Response Testing™, my health had already started improving, but it was very slow. Since doing Nutrition Response Testing™ and Designed Clinical Nutrition, I have seen dramatic changes in areas that were previously stuck.

I do not have sinus issues any more, even during allergy season. I lie down and sleep through the night and wake up refreshed and alert. I can concentrate, focus and process concepts and apply ideas. I can stand for several hours free of pain and tension. My children tell me that they have a healthier mother now than when I was raising them. I have improved so dramatically physically, mentally, and spiritually that I have now the stamina, energy, and skills to operate the business that I own, DayStar Natural, LLC.

My clients are realizing a 90% (or better) improvement in their health and getting results never possible before. To repair the body and restore health is God's ultimate healing. To "Get Healthy and Stay Healthy" with Nutrition Response Testing™ was a divine appointment from God!

I wish that I could convince everyone of the many benefits of having a good nutritional diet, using correct minerals and vitamin supplementation provided by the biofeedback of the body. I realize not everyone will take the courage to step outside the box and brave the unknown phenomena of muscle testing or neurological reflex analysis. I will continue to pursue the techniques that have helped so many achieve their health goals naturally. The following excerpt from "God's Little Devotional Book for Leaders" by W.B. Freeman Concepts, Inc. and Honor Books has been a reminder of why I choose to stay on this course.

My Journey to Health

Do it Anyway

When people are unreasonable, illogical, self-centered, and arrogant, love them anyway.

When people insist that your goodness contains selfish ulterior motives, do good anyway.

If you are successful, you will win both friends and enemies. People may become jealous of you. Succeed anyway.

If you are honest and frank, you will be both honorable and vulnerable. Some will seek to twist your words against you. Be honest and frank anyway.

If you do good today, some may forget about it by tomorrow. Do good anyway.

If you show yourself to be a big person with great ideas, don't be surprised if you are opposed by small people with closed minds. Think big anyway.

What you have spent years building, some may seek to destroy overnight. Build anyway.

Mark Twain once said, "Always do right. This will gratify most people and astonish the rest!"

Kathy Stricker
Board Certified Naturopath

My Journey to Health

CHAPTER 2

Laying the Groundwork

Truthfully, alternative health, natural remedies, and non-invasive techniques can be quite mysterious and appear to be a strange phenomena. I have to admit how I was skeptical at first yet fascinated by the simplicity of healing naturally. I wanted to know more, and the more I pursued the answers, the more my passion was fueled.

Facts based on research:

- 50% of Americans will die from one of the following diseases: diabetes, heart disease, cancer, obesity, and medical bloopers.

- Every cancer diagnosis creates five jobs.

- Heart disease is the leading cause of death in the United States. *National Vital Statistics Report*

- More than one-third of U.S. adults (35.7%) are obese. *NCHS Data Brief No.82, January 2012*

- 1 out of 5 patients is given a completely wrong diagnosis by their doctor. *People's Medical Society*

- Treating cancer is a $115 billion a year business. *National Coalition for Cancer Research*

- 25.8 million children and adults in the United States – 8.3% of the population – have diabetes. *National Diabetes Fact Sheet, 2011*

- Up to 7 out of 10 cancers can be prevented. *American Institute for Cancer Research*

- A recent study found 40 errors a day in the average U.S. hospital. *The Wall Street Journal*

- Each year, over a million hospital patients are injured, and 120,000 die from errors during treatment. *Dr Lucian L. Leape, Harvard medical professor*

Evaluation of Your Health

Stand back and look at yourself in a mirror. Ask yourself these questions honestly, and if you feel you need a little help with this, ask a family member or a trusted friend who will be candid with you. Keep in mind that this person is someone who cares about you and is willing to go the extra mile to help you accomplish your health goals.

Rate each question on a scale of 1-10 (1 is worst, 10 is best).

How would you rate your current health? 4

Is your body strong enough to prevent a serious illness? NO

How would you rate:

- *Your father's health?* Died of canser
- *Your mother's health?* Excellent
- *Your paternal grandmother's health?* heart problems
- *Your paternal grandfather's health?* died of heart attack
- *Your maternal grandmother's health?* died of cancer
- *Your maternal grandfather's health?* Excellent

How fearful are you that you will inherit unhealthy family traits?
Realistically aware

If you scored 30 or less, you need to keep reading this book. What health conditions you would like to overcome?

If you scored 31-65, you have room for improvement. What will your health look like in two years or five years if these conditions do not change?

If you scored 66-100, let's be realistic! Most of us have something to work on. You may be healthy, but you certainly want to learn how to keep your health. Keep reading!

- Do you have plans to get healthy or to stay healthy? *Get*
- Do you want to improve your health within a year, within two years? *ASAP*
- Have you accomplished anything in your life that makes you proud? *No*
- What else would you like to accomplish? *Get healthy*

Without health and the motivation to accomplish your goals, life moves forward slowly, and you never experience all that you were intended to be.

Now for the Basics

The body requires five basic elements to thrive and to survive – oxygen, nutrition, water, heat, and elimination. The Nobel Peace Prize winner Alexis Carrel conducted an experiment in 1912 with his theory that cells are immortal if they are given these five basic elements.

Alexis Carrel kept chicken heart cells alive in a test tube for 34 years. Chickens generally only live three to five years. Every forty-eight hours, the mineralized water that bathed the cells was changed. The cells were always living in a clean, mineral-rich solution. Two years after Carrel's death, the experiment was purposely terminated. *(Natural News, January, 2010)*

The body was designed to be self-healing. It will adapt to any physical or mental situation it faces and responds perfectly.

"For you created my inmost being; you knit me together in my mother's womb." *Psalm 139:13 NIV*

Prevention is our responsibility, which is better than a cure. Our lifestyle choices affect our health.

"Anyone, then, who knows the good he ought to do and doesn't do it, sins." *James 4:17 NIV*

"A minister of the gospel should be a dietician. It is not easy to pray when you suffer from indigestion. It is not easy to be a good Christian when there is acid and poison in the stomach and bowel. A minister should tell his congregation what to eat." *The Chemistry of Man, Bernard Jensen, 1983*

"Don't you know that you yourselves are God's temple and that God's Spirit lives in you? If anyone destroys God's temple, God will destroy him; for God's temple is sacred, and you are that temple." "You are not your own; you were bought at a price. Therefore honor God with your body." *I Cor. 3:16-17, I Cor. 6:20 NIV*

Psychologists claim that it takes 21 days to form a new habit. It will take time, determination, and a coach to help you regain your health. Although it may feel like you are pushing a huge two-ton locomotive by yourself at first, in time your efforts will pay off, and you will look back in retrospect with gratitude and thanksgiving that you made the first step to getting your health back.

"Everyone who competes in the games goes into strict training. They do it to get a crown that will not last; but we do it to get a crown that will last forever. Therefore, I do not run like a man running aimlessly; I do not fight like a man beating the air. No, I beat my body and make it my slave so that after I have preached to others, I myself will not be disqualified for the prize."
I Corinthians 9:25-27 NIV

Let's Start that Strict Training with Weight Loss Tips!

Millions of people are looking for an easy way to lose weight. If you attempt to go on a diet or improve your eating habits, you may cave when hunger kicks in or when you smell something cooking or simply give up in frustration. The following suggestions will help you make wiser choices and encourage you to keep on the right track.

Curb your cravings with an apple or celery with raw almond butter.

- When you see, smell, or dwell on food, you are more likely to give in to cravings. Drive past a fast food restaurant or a doughnut shop, and the smell in the air will cause you to feel hungry. If you wait about 20 minutes or drink something warm like a cup of hot tea, the cravings usually stop.

- Water will make you feel fuller but without the calories. Hunger cravings are often mistaken for dehydration. One glass of water first thing in the morning is highly beneficial.

- Brush your teeth and smell some anise, fennel, or vanilla.

- Sometimes nothing else works like biting into a dessert or sugary food. Take only one bite, and let it slowly melt in your mouth. If you are like me, you may notice that the treat does not taste as good as it did before.

Finally, here is one fact that will have you thinking. One pound of body fat is equal to 3500 calories. So, to lose a pound a week, reduce 500 calories per day. You may want to rethink that McDonald's Quarter Pounder® with Cheese (520 calories), a Premium Crispy Chicken Classic Sandwich (510 calories), Large French Fries (500 calories) or that Bacon, Egg & Cheese Biscuit (520 calories). Just saying!

CHAPTER 3

Letting Go

The following story is from a book I had read somewhere. I wanted to give credit to the author, but I could not find the correct resource. Even researching the internet, the story was told differently, and no author was referenced.

The Necklace

The cheerful little girl with bouncy golden curls was almost five. Waiting with her mother at the checkout stand, she saw them, a circle of glistening white pearls in a pink foil box.

"Oh mommy please, Mommy. Can I have them? Please, Mommy, please?"

Quickly the mother checked the back of the little foil box and then looked back into the pleading blue eyes of her little girl's upturned face.

"A dollar ninety-five. That's almost $2.00. If you really want them, I'll think of some extra chores for you, and in no time, you can save enough money to buy them for yourself. Your birthday's only a week away, and you might get another crisp dollar bill from Grandma."

As soon as Jenny got home, she emptied her penny bank and counted out 17 pennies. After dinner, she did more than her share of chores, and she went to the neighbor and asked Mrs. McJames if she could pick dandelions for ten cents. On her birthday, Grandma did give her another new dollar bill, and at last, she had enough money to buy the necklace.

Jenny loved her pearls. They made her feel dressed up and grown up. She wore them everywhere, Sunday school, kindergarten, even to bed. The only time she took them off was when she went swimming or had a bubble bath. Mother said if they got wet, they might turn her neck green.

Jenny had a very caring father, and every night when she was ready for bed, he would stop whatever he was doing and come upstairs to read her a story. One night as he finished the story, he asked Jenny, "Do you love me?"

"Oh yes, daddy. You know that I love you."

"Then give me your pearls."

"Oh, daddy, not my pearls. But you can have Princess, the white horse from my collection, the one with the pink tail. Remember, daddy? The one you gave me. She's my very favorite."

"That's okay, Honey, daddy loves you. Good night." And he brushed her cheek with a kiss.

About a week later, after the story time, Jenny's daddy asked again, "Do you love me?"

"Daddy, you know I love you."

"Then give me your pearls."

"Oh Daddy, not my pearls. But you can have my baby doll. The brand new one I got for my birthday. She is beautiful, and you can have the yellow blanket that matches her sleeper."

"That's okay. Sleep well. God bless you, little one. Daddy loves you." And as always, he brushed her cheek with a gentle kiss.

A few nights later when her daddy came in, Jenny was sitting on her bed with her legs crossed Indian style.

As he came close, he noticed her chin was trembling, and one silent tear rolled down her cheek.

"What is it, Jenny? What's the matter?"

Jenny didn't say anything but lifted her little hand up to her daddy. And when she opened it, there was her little pearl necklace. With a little quiver, she finally said, "Here, daddy; this is for you."

With tears gathering in his own eyes, Jenny's daddy reached out with one hand to take the dime store necklace, and with the other hand, he reached into his pocket and pulled out a blue velvet case with a strand of genuine pearls and gave them to Jenny.

He had them all the time. He was just waiting for her to give up the dime-store stuff so he could give her the genuine treasure. So it is, with our Heavenly Father. He is waiting for us to give up the cheap things in our lives so that he can give us beautiful treasures.

Are you holding on to relationships, habits, and activities that you have become so attached to that it seems impossible to let go? In spite of what you cannot see, trust that God will never take away something from you without giving you something better in its place.

"Again, the kingdom of heaven is like a merchant looking for fine pearls. When he found one of great value, he went away and sold everything he had and bought it." *Matthew 13:45-46 NIV*

"Do not be wise in your own eyes; fear the LORD, and shun evil. This will bring health to your body and nourishment to your bones." *Proverbs 3: 7-8 NIV*

Symptoms are a physical evidence of poor nutrition in the body. Organs need good nutrition to perform, function, and support the demands on the body. The roots of disease are poor nutrition and unhealthy lifestyles.

PMS, Menopause, Hot Flashes, Irritability, Heavy Bleeding

Allergies, Asthma Bronchitis Sinus Infections

Arthritis, Osteopenia, Osteoporosis, Gout, Degenerative Disk Disease

Crohn's Disease, GERD Indigestion, Constipation, Diarrhea, Diverticulitis

Diabetes Hypoglycemia Weight Gain

ADD/ADHD Autism Learning Disabilities Behavioral Disorders

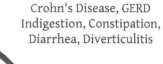
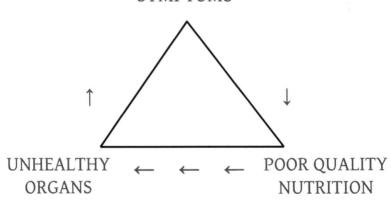

SYMPTOMS

UNHEALTHY ORGANS ← ← ← POOR QUALITY NUTRITION

"Patients indeed have played a strong role in choosing their diseases (cancer, heart disease, back disease, arthritis, and chronic respiratory illness)... by smoking, overeating, and not exercising, which aggravate the diseases." *Dr. Bruce R. Zimmerman of the Mayo Clinic, September 20, 2005*

"They acquire these conditions as the chemical elements are depleted from their body." *The Chemistry of Man, 1983, Bernard Jensen, PhD*

Letting Go

CHAPTER 4

Body Systems
and
Functions

Five fundamentals to health are spelled out in the acrostic "CLEAN": a clean **C**olon, take time for **L**eisure, get **E**xercise, have a great **A**ttitude, and get proper **N**utrition. Understanding pH levels is one of the first steps towards preserving the five fundamentals.

pH is the degree of acidity and alkalinity of a solution. pH is measured on a logarithmic scale of 1 to 14. Anything with a pH value of less than 7.0 is considered acidic. Anything with a pH of greater than 7.0 is considered alkaline.

Saliva pH should be from 6.0 to 7.0 (mildly acid to neutral). Urine pH should be from 4.5 to 8.0 (somewhat acid to slightly alkaline). Over a 24-hour period, pH levels change. Urine is slightly more acid in the morning (pH=6.4-7.0) and by evening, becomes more alkaline (pH=7.5-8.0).

Human cells are like fish in an aquarium. They are susceptible to disease or death when the fluids are not in a perfect pH environment. If the pH range of the cells becomes too acidic, then the tissues become toxic.

Poor nutrition cannot alkalize the tissues but will make it more difficult to remove toxic wastes. The colon will back up, and acid waste will be dumped back into the blood stream and organs. More acid will be accumulated, and the body will slowly degenerate.

You may be one of those people who say you can eat anything, that you have an "iron" stomach. Or you may have recognized the upset to your digestive tract after eating and have commented, "I wish I hadn't eaten that."

Those "warnings" are your body talking to you. If you ignore the signals, illness will be lurking, and your health will be like a bomb waiting to go off. For some people, the integrity of the body is comprised of such strong constitution that it may take years of nutritional abuse before symptoms are manifested.

Destructive acid pH imbalance impacts the kidneys, liver, pancreas, gall bladder, and all bodily functions that depend on those organs. Gout, ulcers, colitis, acid reflux, blemishes and acne, cancer, immune system deficiencies, and neurological dysfunction are just a few symptoms that can occur.

Everything you put into your mouth that enters the digestive system has a pH value. Protein animal products such as meat, poultry, eggs, and dairy are considered low pH foods. Simple and complex carbohydrates like processed foods made from white refined sugar and white flour (cake, cookies, candy, ice cream, pastries, etc.) have a low pH value. Coffee, tea, wine, soda, prescription drugs, and artificial sweeteners (NutraSweet®, Equal®, Aspartame, Splenda®) have an even lower pH.

When essential alkaline electrolytes and soluble minerals are missing in the kidneys to buffer and neutralize the low acidic pH, the body robs nutrients from the bones, cells, and tissues. It is this nutrient deficiency that causes disease and premature aging.

For 5-10 days, pass a strip of pH test paper through a stream of urine, and then match the color with the test kit. The first morning urine will give a picture of the internal environment. Most of us will test acid due to poor nutrition, stressful lifestyles, and lack of exercise.

The next step to understanding your body is to know where the organs are and how the body systems function. The following descriptions are very simple. For details, there is a vast amount of information available today, which can easily be found online.

The Circulatory System

Your heart is your strongest muscle. It pumps the blood throughout the body. Although the heart is only about the size of your fist, it beats about 3 billion times during an average lifetime.

The circulatory system functions to receive nutrition, replenish oxygen, and remove waste to over 100 trillion cells throughout the body. The blood is the transportation medium composed of red and white blood cells, plasma, and platelets.

Arteries are the thick vessels that carry blood away from the heart, and veins carry blood to the heart. Capillaries are the tiny vessels that connect the arteries to the veins throughout the whole body, but amazingly, some capillaries are only the width of a single blood cell.

The average human body has four to six liters of blood. Red blood cells are made in the bone marrow and live for about 120 days. Old red cells are eventually destroyed in the liver or spleen. An average of 2.5 million red blood cells are destroyed per second!

Blood is circulated around the body more than 1,000 times per day. That's five to six thousand quarts of blood pumped by your heart every day, and each drop contains about 5 million red blood cells.

White blood cells attack and destroy germs when they enter the body. When you have an infection, your body will produce more white blood cells. Platelets are blood cells that help stop bleeding. Platelets stick to the opening of damaged vessels attracting more platelets, fibers, and other blood cells and form a plug (scab) to seal the broken blood vessel.

Plasma is the liquid component of blood and circulates everything throughout the body. Plasma has a clear to yellowish color and is comprised of about 90% water.

When the body is in an excess acid status, viruses can attach themselves to the inner wall of arteries and cause plaque to form in the artery. With this restriction of the flow of blood, oxygen, and nutrients, a heart attack may occur. Calcium deposits on plaque and makes the arteries stiff and raise blood pressure.

To support the circulatory system, it is important to make dietary changes. Fruits and vegetables contain the amounts of vitamins and minerals the body needs to function. Use sea salt to replenish the sodium (alkaline) reserves in a form that is easily assimilated.

Salt and sodium are not the same. Table salt is an active element of sodium and chloride, which the body cannot break down into a usable form. The body needs an organic form of sodium, such as Pink Salt (Premier Research Labs).

Some fast food restaurants may have as much as 1,000 mg of sodium in a burger; twenty french fries may have 100 mg; 300 mg for a chocolate shake; and 1,200-1,800 mg of sodium for half of a 14-inch frozen pizza. The average American consumes 5,000 mg of sodium per day.

When preparing foods, experiment with a few of the culinary herbs, such as rosemary, basil, mint, oregano, tarragon, thyme, cumin, curry, or cayenne. Sesame, anise, coriander, and mustard seeds are also good for adding a little flavor. Avoid using lemon pepper, fajita seasoning, meat tenderizer, bouillon cubes, or other "flavorings", as these may contain salt or monosodium glutamate (MSG), a known toxin.

The Nervous System

Your brain, spinal column, and all the nerves of the body make up the nervous system. The pituitary, hypothalamus, pineal gland, and cerebellum are responsible for every thought, emotion, and action.

Walking, breathing, and thinking all result from the activity of the nervous system. Billions of nerve cells respond to and process information and send out electrical signals, which travel more than 200 miles per hour. The nerves are small, yet they are most complex and versatile.

When the body is too acidic, it is unable to produce chemicals called neurotransmitters. Symptoms such as insomnia, anxiety, depression, neuroses, psychoses, and impairment of memory are the result. Pure therapeutic grade essential oils of lavender, bergamot, sandalwood, and blue chamomile will penetrate cell walls to relax and calm the nervous system.

The Structural/Skeletal System

Bones are the living, growing, changing structure of the body that make up our framework. Without our bones, we would be like jellyfish! We are born with around 270 bones, but by the time we become adults, we only have 206 since the baby bones made of cartilage are slowly replaced by harder bone.

Interesting facts about bones:

- Bones protect the softer parts of our bodies.
- The skull is like a natural helmet that protects the brain.
- The spine protects all the nerves in the spinal column.
- The ribs make a shield around our lungs, heart, and liver.
- Bones are hard on the outside and soft but strong on the inside.
- Red and white blood cells are made inside bones from bone marrow.
- Bones are made of protein called collagen, vitamins, minerals, and calcium.
- Calcium stored in the bones is released in order to neutralize excess acid in the tissues.
- Muscle cramps, osteoporosis, poor back posture, back pain, and degenerative arthritis are related to calcium deficiencies, and magnesium assists in the assimilation of calcium.
- Walking, climbing, and dancing are exercises that make bones strong and healthy.
- Weight bearing exercises help build or maintain bone.
- Fresh fruit and vegetables help to alkalize the bones.

The Digestive System

The body will try to digest what we put into our mouths by the process known as peristalsis – the progressive wave of contraction and relaxation of the alimentary canal to propel food from the mouth to the rectum.

The glands of the digestive system produce enzymes responsible for digestion. Small amounts of saliva, gastric juice, pancreatic juice, bile, and intestinal juice are constantly secreted by these glands as food travels from the mouth, through the esophagus, and into the stomach where it mixes with these juices, forming a soup-like substance.

Gastric bypass surgery, performed as a method of weight reduction, eliminates some of the secretions necessary for proper digestion. As the food continues on into the small intestine, juices from the liver mix with this thick substance, and the useful components are extracted and sent into the blood where they are needed.

Once the food goes to the large intestine, it combines with water from the food and goes into the blood. At this point, the body has taken everything it can use from the food. Waste will be stored inside the rectum until muscles push the waste out.

DIGESTION AND TIME FRAMES

Mouth – Voluntary

From the moment food is placed in the mouth, peristalsis starts the process of assimilation, digestion, and elimination.

Carbohydrates digestion begins in the mouth. Chew your food 30-50 times per bite, and take stress off of the other organs of digestion.

The tip of the tongue is the center for sweet tastes. No wonder we have a sugar addiction. We have become an obese nation, overfed and undernourished.

"The human tongue is physically small. It can poison the whole body." *James 3:8 KJV*

"All man's efforts are for his mouth, yet his appetite is never satisfied." *Ecclesiastes 6:7 NIV*

A few years ago, an anonymous writer submitted a parody on God's and Satan's view of food. It goes like this:

> "In the beginning, God created the Heavens and the earth, and populated the earth with broccoli and cauliflower and spinach; green and yellow and red vegetables of all kinds so Man and Woman would live long and healthy lives. And Satan created McDonald's, and man underwent cardiac arrest. Then God created a light, fluffy white cake, named it 'Angel Food', and said 'It is good!' Then Satan created chocolate cake and named it 'Devil's Food'."

How true it is that we are controlled by our taste buds. The road to good health is an upward journey, and at the end of the road is a healthy body. Only you can make the decision to become a catalyst for change from sickness and disease to health and abundant living.

Pharynx – less than 1 second

Esophagus – 10 seconds

Stomach – 3 to 4 hours

- The stomach is flat until food expands the muscle.
- The stomach produces HCl (hydrochloric acid) to digest protein.
- Proteins are broken down into amino acids in the stomach.
- Carbohydrate digestion is completed in the stomach.
- Fat digestion begins in the stomach.
- pH is extremely acidic – 2.0.

Small Intestine – up to 5 hours

The function of the small intestine is to digest and absorb nutrients from the food particles that arrive from the stomach.

Large Intestine – 12 to 36 hours

(ascending, transverse, and descending colon)

The large intestines are the holding tank for toxins. When elimination is sluggish or constipation occurs, the blood stream becomes toxic as it reabsorbs undigested fermentation and putrefaction. The bowels can hold excessive populations of unfriendly microorganisms such as bacteria, viruses, parasites, and fungi (yeasts, candida albicans). Bad breath often is an indication of poor bowel movements.

Rectum

This is last stage in the process of peristalsis represented in an urge to release toxic waste.

The digestive tract is 18 to 27 feet long. The liver, pancreas, and gallbladder are included in the digestive system but are not part of the digestive tract. Nausea, vomiting, celiac disease, food intolerance, hernias, gallstones, ulcers, gas, and bloating are manifestations of digestive distress.

ALEXIS ST. MARTIN'S STORY

Excerpts from "Biologic Ionization As Applied to Human Nutrition", A.F. Beddoe, June 2002

"From 1825 to 1835, William Beaumont, a young surgeon with the U.S. Army, treated Alexis St. Martin, an 18 year old Canadian, for a shotgun blast at three foot range. As a result of the accident, parts of his inner body were exposed. These openings healed peripherally and were closed internally by a 'flap valve' of tissue (the actual inner coats of the stomach), which could be pushed aside, enabling ready access and direct view of the stomach."

"St. Martin recovered, and Beaumont performed innumerable digestion experiments on him for ten years. Beaumont would insert a tube through the hole into the stomach several times each week and draw off about 1½ ounces of 'pure gastric juice'. Beaumont showed that gastric juice, either in the stomach or outside in a test tube, will break down foodstuffs in from 1 to 4 hours."

"Stomach emptying time showed a dependence on the type of food, as well as to how well the food was chewed. This points out how important it is to chew each mouthful extremely well to help the stomach. If it is not masticated well, the speed of stomach emptying is affected. This is one main contributor to indigestion."

"Beaumont: 'Improper indulgence in eating and drinking has been the most common precursor of these diseased conditions of the coats of the stomach. The free use of ardent spirits, wine, beer, or any intoxicating liquor, when continued for some days, has invariably produced these morbid changes. I would concur that improper eating (including poor quality food) and drinking in the lifestyle of the individual are the biggest single contributing factors to degenerative disease.'"

GASTRIC BYPASS AND RISKS

When I first opened my doors for business, a woman in her early 40's asked for help. The regime of vitamins, supplements, and medications suggested by her doctor after gastric bypass surgery was not working for her.

She was losing her hearing, her eyesight was failing, and she could not absorb nutrients. Since I was teaching classes on health at that time, she begged me to share her experience with everyone. She sensed that she was losing the battle and requested that my husband (a pastor) perform her funeral service. Her symptoms worsened, and she passed away a few months later.

Gastric bypass surgeries create a small stomach pouch to restrict food intake and bypass the duodenum and other segments of the small intestine, which causes malabsorption (decreased ability to absorb nutrients from food).

According to study results reported in the Journal of the American Medical Association, 2% (one in every 50) gastric bypass surgery patients died within 30 days of the operations. Almost 5% (one in 20) died within a year. Complications range from infections, incisional hernias, ulcers, blood clots in the lungs, internal leaking, and peritonitis.

Patients who make it through the operation may benefit from improvements in common obesity-related health issues such as diabetes, heart disease, and lung function.

Researchers studied 66,109 obese patients. The first group consisted of 3,328 patients who received gastric bypass surgery while the second group included the remainder of the patients or those hospitalized for some other medical reason.

In the time span of 30 days, one in 50 surgery patients died (almost 67 people). Approximately 3% (about 100 people) of patients who had gastric bypass surgery were younger than 40 and died after 13.6 years, compared to the 13.8% who did not have the surgery. After 15 years, 11.8% (366 people) of patients of all ages who had gastric bypass surgery died, compared to the 16.3% who did not have the surgery.

An important note: The success rate of gastric bypass surgery reflects the experience of the surgeon – patients are at up to a five times greater risk of death during surgery if the surgeon is less experienced.

The Intestinal System

The intestinal system extends from the stomach to the anus and includes the small and large intestines. The small intestine is involved with the digestion and assimilation of food. The large intestine is involved in the storage and disposal of waste material.

The large intestine is divided into the cecum, the ascending colon, the transverse colon, the descending colon, the sigmoid colon, the rectum, and the anus.

Testing the pH of the saliva can indicate the activity of the liver and stomach enzymes. Salivary pH should be between 6.4 – 6.8. Diarrhea, irritable bowel syndrome, colitis, inflammatory bowel disease (Crohn's), hemorrhoids, constipation, or diverticulitis are symptoms related to the pH imbalances of the intestinal system.

Diarrhea Relief: One capsule of activated charcoal taken every hour until symptoms subside (but no more than three days).

Irritable bowel: Peppermint oil rubbed on the abdomen to alleviate pain. Although it sounds too simple, many problems of the intestinal system can be helped by chewing food 30 or more times with each bite of food.

COLON FACTS

Managing bowel habits is one of the most important steps to protect your health. A toxic colon comes from the accumulation of undigested food rotting in the gut or parasites stealing your food and poisoning your body with their wastes.

"Death begins in the colon." *Ascribed to Dr. Bernard Jensen, D.C., referred to as the "Father of Colonics"*

- The digestive system and colon health have reached an all-time low in the U.S.
- In 1994 the #1 cancer was in the colon.
- A colon should move 2 if not 3 times a day.
- A clean colon is necessary for the health of the whole human.
- When our colon is distorted, scarred, plugged, twisted, and lined with old material (sometimes days or weeks old), putrefying and hosting parasites, it makes us feel sluggish.

To make matters worse, this sewage has a way of seeping into the blood stream, and we begin to circulate our own old stinky wastes through our bodies. This makes us look and feel sick; hence, "death begins in the colon."

- When our colon is plugged, our brain cannot function correctly.

- When our colon needs attention and does not work properly, it causes a complete chain reaction of events to occur. The liver loses it's power to create the proper enzymes and acids to digest food, and so our digestive system slows down, which in turn, may create pancreatic problems, then causing blood sugar and thyroid problems.

- A potbelly is a sign of toxemia, commercial food backed up, and severe putrefaction.

- Over time everyone with a toxic colon will get a toxic liver. Degenerative disease comes from a toxic liver, which comes from a toxic colon.

- Laxatives often irritate the colon, and after a time of regular use, they quit working, too.

- There is no quick fix or magic pill that will cure a problematic colon, but this is what people want.

- Lack of sufficient water and too much refined foods (white flour, white sugar, etc.) and not enough of fiber in the diet causes colon toxicity.

- Prolonged stress causes the colon to sag in the middle, creating a trap for material to stay there and putrefy.

- Fiber from raw vegetables prevents undigested food from sticking to the colon.

- Knox gelatin daily with prune juice and millet, okra, olive oil, and flax seeds are wonderful colon foods.

- If people take deep massage enemas (colonics), they do not need an appendix operation.

- Diverticulitis is caused by too much salt in the lining of the intestines that causes pockets, and the food lodges there, and the only way to get it out is through deep massage enemas (colonics).

- A pear a day keeps a colon healthy.

- The best way to support the lungs is to cleanse the colon with deep massage enemas (colonics) and essential oils.

- Deep massage enemas (colonics) give your colon flexibility and opens up the little fingers that absorb nutrients as well as loosens and expels old impacted fecal material.

- A variety of essential oils with deep massage enemas (colonics) will kill parasites, reduce inflammation of the colon, digest toxins, poisons, and chemicals. They will help facilitate the proper healing of a colon and help restore it into balance.

"In the 50 years I've spent helping people to overcome illness, disability, and disease, it has become crystal clear that poor bowel management lies at the root of most people's health problems. In treating over 300,000 patients, it is the bowel that invariably has to be cared for before any healing can take place." *Dr. Bernard Jensen, PhD*

The Liver

The largest gland in the body is the liver and maintains health through more than 500 functions. It is located on the right, below the ribs, weighs about three pounds, and is approximately eight inches long. The liver stores glycogen, a form of glucose that is used as energy when levels fall between meals. The liver manufactures vitamin A and stores vitamins D, K, and B_{12}.

The liver receives blood and converts the nutrients into usable products for the body. It plays a major role in metabolism, digestion, and elimination of toxic substances. It is vital to have a healthy liver.

Alcohol, drugs, bacteria, and old blood cells are broken down and removed from the body in the liver. If the liver is busy processing toxic chemicals, its functions are limited. Therefore, cleansing the liver is important.

LIVER DETOX

Use as much as you want of pure apple juice (no high fructose corn syrup or other sugar additives), or throw in a few apples. Drink before going to bed for five consecutive days.

In a blender combine:

1 banana, peeled

1 lemon, peeled and cut into quarters

1 handful of parsley

1 clove garlic

1 small piece of ginger root

1 tablespoon first cold-pressed olive oil

The Gallbladder

The gallbladder, a small sac on the underside of the right lobe of the liver, stores bile that is made by the liver. It holds about two ounces of bile, which breaks down the fat in food.

If in doubt, consult with your physician before using the following flushes or enemas.

GALLBLADDER FLUSH TECHNIQUE

This procedure assists the removal of concretions from the gallbladder. For five days, consume 1 quart of raw apple juice each day. Cut the hard fats out of the diet, and use lots of raw and cooked fruits. On the evening of the 5th day, just before bed, mix ½ cup of fresh lemon juice and ½ cup of first-cold pressed olive oil. Drink the lemon and olive oil mixture at bedtime; go to bed, place a heating pad over the liver area (right side under rib cage) while lying on the right side. Sleep in this position. Upon arising in the morning, drink another ½ cup of lemon juice and ½ cup olive oil mixture. Wait two hours, and take the coffee enema. A plain tap water enema is recommended prior to the coffee enema.

PLAIN WATER HIGH ENEMA

This is done by introducing plain tap water into the lower colon while being in a knee-chest position. In a knee chest position, kneel on the floor then bend over until knees are almost touching the chest. The buttocks will be up in the air so that the colon is lower than the rectum. As the water is introduced into the colon, the elimination response in this pose is less. This type of enema is done with a coffee enema following it, separated by 15 minutes of rest. This is so that the fecal material that is loosened by the first is always voided with the second in the procedure.

COFFEE ENEMA

Coffee enemas stimulate the dilation of the gallbladder and bile ducts to help eliminate waste from the liver into the colon. The solution is made with three tablespoons of ground organic coffee in two quarts of water. Boil the coffee and water for 10 minutes, then cool until only moderately warm. Filter the solution and, pour it into an enema bucket. Apply sesame oil to the tip of the tube, and place an old towel in the bathtub or on the floor to lie on. Raise the bucket approximately two feet above the rectum, and lie on your back while you insert the tube into the rectum. Release the clamp to allow the warm solution to flow. It is best to start with 8 ounces and hold the coffee solution as long as possible. A 5 to 10 minute hold will help to get the full effect of the contraction response. Do as many 8 ounce holds as possible, and gradually increase the amount to 18 to 28 ounces, based on your comfort level.

The Pancreas

The pancreas is below the stomach. The pancreas produces glucagon and supplies insulin. Glucagon and insulin regulate and balance blood sugar. It also produces and releases enzymes to assist in digestion.

Enzymes to the body are like money in the bank. When the withdrawals are greater than the supply, you go broke. The pancreas will supply enzymes as long as it can. Unless we make changes to ensure enzymes are there when needed, the source will become exhausted.

Rubbing pure, therapeutic-grade essential oil of peppermint on the abdomen will help. However, the best solution is to stop using antacids and to thoroughly chew your food between 30 and 50 chews each bite. Antacids neutralize hydrochloric acid. You need hydrochloric acid to break down proteins because undigested proteins can cause pain and inflammation. The stomach should be very acidic (pH of 2.0).

HOW TO INCREASE ENZYMES

First, make wiser food choices. Eat more raw foods. Steam or cook foods with lower heat. Take a supplement that includes protease, amylase, and lipase with meals to help reduce excess acid and support digestion.

Extra virgin olive oil, raw honey, grapes, figs, avocados, dates, bananas, papaya, pineapple, kiwi, and mangoes have high enzyme contents. Grains, nuts, legumes, and seeds are also rich in enzymes; however, they also contain enzyme inhibitors.

Enzyme inhibitors protect seeds from germinating prematurely but can slow down digestion more than cooked foods. Sprouting and soaking in warm water help deactivate enzyme inhibitors. Potatoes, eggs, and especially raw peanuts also have enzyme inhibitors.

Frying robs foods of natural enzymes. Microwaving alters the molecular structure of foods and destroys enzymes. Long term use of over-the-counter acid blockers upsets the delicate balance of friendly bacteria and enzymes, which can inhibit the ability to break down food and get rid of waste.

A safer solution to calm heartburn and upset stomachs is to use peppermint essential oil topically. One drop rubbed on the tummy, penetrates the skin and effectively works to reduce digestive distress.

The Immune System

The immune system is complex because there is more than one organ involved. The thymus, spleen, lymph system, bone marrow, white blood cells, antibodies, and hormones all work together to clear infection from the body and to defend you against bacteria, microbes, viruses, toxins, and parasites.

Your skin is the first wall of protection against foreign invaders that cause disease. Our skin renews itself every 28 days, sloughing off old, dead skin cells and replacing them with fresh new ones.

The second line of defense is fluids, like mucus, found in your respiratory system, and tears from your eyes. If the invaders do pass through these defenses, the next line are the white blood cells to fight the germs. They are probably the most important part of your immune system.

Blood plasma, or lymph, is a transparent fluid that bathes the cells and tissues of the body with water and nutrients. Fluids ooze into the lymphatic system and get pushed by normal body and muscle motion to the lymph nodes. There is no "lymph pump" like there is a "blood pump" (the heart). Exercise is the pump. Get moving!

Inflammation and pus are both side effects of the immune system doing its job. Fevers, hives, inflammation, colds, influenza, measles, mumps, malaria, cancer and AIDS, Juvenile-onset diabetes, rheumatoid arthritis, and allergies are some of the many symptoms that indicate the immune system is making an attempt to do its job.

Restrictive clothing prevents the flow of blood and lymph. Wearing a bra to prevent sagging breasts actually weakens the muscles and connective tissue helping to create sagging breasts. The free movement of the breasts during walking and exercise helps to pump lymph through the breast tissue.

Peppermint and elderberry tea are good for colds. Climb stairs, walk to the store, ride a bicycle, use a push mower to cut the grass, plant a garden, go for a walk after dinner each day. When you are active physically, you are assisting your cells in the clearing of toxins.

Do not overeat; it suppresses the immune system. Cell repair work takes place while you are sleeping, and the average sleep requirement is nine hours. An hour of sleep before midnight is worth two hours after, because the circadian rhythm of the body dictates when each organ will function at its best – when to heal and when to clean.

Rebounding is a great exercise for the immune system. For more information on rebounding, see page 191.

The Respiratory System

The respiratory system is made of the trachea, the lungs, and the diaphragm. You breathe in oxygen and exhale carbon dioxide. The trachea, or windpipe, is the tube that carries the air from the mouth or nose. It divides into two sections called the bronchi.

Oxygen enters the lungs, passing through a spongy structure containing a network of blood vessels. These blood vessels bring carbon dioxide to the lungs for removal and transport oxygen from the lungs to the rest of the body.

Breathing is subconscious. When breathing in, muscles lift the ribs up and forward while the diaphragm moves downward to expand the lungs. When breathing out, muscles and the diaphragm relax, and air is pushed out and up through the trachea.

Bronchitis, pneumonia, sinusitis, cough, bronchial spasms (asthma), allergies, and hay fever are respiratory imbalances. Remedies for the immune system will also apply for the respiratory system as well. For asthma attacks, inhale pure therapeutic grade essential oil of lavender.

Urinary System

The urinary system – the kidneys, ureters, bladder, and urethra – regulates the concentrations of various electrolytes in the body fluids.

The urinary system keeps chemicals and water in balance and maintains normal pH of the blood. Urinary pH levels indicate how well your body is assimilating minerals, especially calcium, magnesium, sodium, and potassium. These minerals are buffers to control acid. Urinary pH should fluctuate between 6.0-6.4 in the morning and 6.4-7.0 in the evening.

The urinary system removes urea, a type of waste, from the blood-stream to the kidneys. Urea is produced when foods containing protein such as meat, poultry, and certain vegetables, are broken down in the body. When acid levels increase, the body stores the acid in the tissues and will borrow minerals from organs and bones in order to neutralize the acids.

Normal urine is sterile and contains fluids, salts, and waste products. It is free of bacteria, viruses, and fungi. Adults pass about one and a half quarts each day, depending on the fluids and foods consumed.

Women have some bacteria or fungi in the bladder. Pain or burning when urinating indicates the reserves of the neutralizing minerals are exhausted and the body has adapted for survival, not comfort. Kidney stones are also an imbalance of the urinary system.

Alleviate pain or burning by drinking several glasses of pure unsweetened cranberry juice a day for a few days. Drink an 8 oz. glass of water every hour. Eat leafy green vegetables, and drink green powder mixes – foods that will replenish the supply of neutralizing minerals.

The Endocrine System

The glands of the endocrine system are small and located throughout the body. They include the thyroid, parathyroid, pituitary, adrenal, hypothalamus, pineal, pancreas, and reproductive glands. Some come in pairs such as the thyroid and adrenal glands.

Endocrine glands release more than 20 major hormones directly into the bloodstream where they can be transported to cells in other parts of the body. Hormones regulate metabolism, growth and development, tissue function, and moods.

When the endocrine glands cannot produce and release sufficient hormones, blood sugar imbalances, fatigue, reproductive difficulties, and mood swings occur. Therapeutic grade essential oils, dietary changes, and stress management therapy are all helpful.

THYROID GLANDS

The thyroid is one of the largest endocrine glands and is located in the front of the neck at the base of the larynx. Its primary function is to stimulate and maintain hormones. There are three hormones produced by the thyroid. A dysfunctional thyroid is often diagnosed medically as hyperthyroidism or hypothyroidism.

Common symptoms of hypothyroidism are brittle fingernails and hair, fatigue, paleness, muscle cramps, and joint pain. Common symptoms of hyperthyroidism are excessive weight loss, anxiety, fatigue, hair loss, weakness, hyperactivity, and irritability.

Thyroid hormones stimulate growth and maturation during child development as well as increased mental activity. The T3 and T4 hormones play a role in the maintenance of normal blood pressure, heart rate, muscle tone, digestion, and reproductive functions.

Other symptoms exhibited by thyroid problems are a racing heart, sensitivity to cold or heat, weight loss or gain, increase or decrease in bowel movements, muscle weakness or spasms, warm, moist skin or cold, dry skin, frequent staring, change in menstrual cycles, insomnia, fatigue, depression, memory problems, and irritability.

PARATHYROID GLANDS

The main function of the parathyroid glands is to regulate calcium in the blood and bones. Calcium allows conduction of the body's nervous system to contribute support from the brain to the rest of the body.

A tingling sensation in fingers or cramps in the muscles indicates a drop in calcium levels. Feeling brain fog or weird sensations, insomnia or restless sleep, feeling run down, lack of energy, depression, irritability, and memory lapses are related to too much or too little calcium.

PINEAL GLAND

The pineal gland is a complex system that plays an important role in physiological and psychological functions of the body. Philosophers and spiritual buffs believe that the pineal gland is where our soul lies. It is referred to as the "third eye" acting as a mediator between the physical and spiritual world.

Melatonin is secreted by the pineal gland. Darkness stimulates the gland to release melatonin, and the light inhibits it. Jet lag, poor vision, and working the third shift can affect melatonin production. Sunlight, light exercise, meditation, and following natural day and night light patterns prevent pineal dysfunctions.

Signals sent by the pineal gland help the body feel thirst and hunger. The pineal gland supplies hormones for sexual desires. Along with the hypothalamus, the pineal gland dictates the body's biological clock and controls the aging process.

PITUITARY GLAND

Located at the base of the brain, the pituitary gland is pea-sized and is referred to as the "master gland". The pituitary gland secretes nine hormones to regulate other organs and endocrine glands, which control our temperature, thyroid activity, growth during childhood, and urine production. The pituitary gland also secretes endorphins that act on the nervous system to reduce pain.

HYPOTHALAMUS GLAND

One function of the hypothalamus is to connect the central nervous system to the endocrine system. The hypothalamus also regulates hormonal and behavioral patterns for seasonal rhythms as well as increase and cessation of food intake. The biological temporal rhythms such as daily (circadian*), weekly, seasonal, and annual rhythms, are adjusted by daylight.

ADRENAL GLANDS

The adrenal glands are small and sit on top of the kidneys. They manufacture several important hormones such as norepinephrine and epinephrine, cortisol, estrogen and testosterone.

Norepinephrine and epinephrine regulate the "fight or flight" response to stressful events. Epinephrine (adrenaline) increases blood pressure and heart rate when stressed. Cortisol regulates the ability to fight off histamines from allergens and minimizes swelling and inflammation from asthma, allergies, and autoimmune disorders.

Caffeine and sugar consumed in excess can lead to symptoms of poor adrenal function such as fatigue, muscle aches, salt and sugar cravings, feeling dehydrated, and periods of insomnia or difficulty falling asleep, which results in irritability and depression. Common food allergies are wheat, eggs, milk, and soy.

There are natural techniques to support the endocrine system such as stress management therapy, dietary changes, and essential

---

* "A circadian rhythm is any biological process that displays an endogenous, entrainable oscillation of about 24 hours." w*ikipedia.org*

oils of lavender, bergamot, and geranium. Hormone balance is important for both men and women.

For PMS relief, work on eliminating omega-6 fatty acids. Boost omega-3 fatty acid levels using cod liver oil, fish, grass-fed, free-range beef, free-range poultry, walnuts, and flax seeds. It may take three to four months for cramps to subside and disappear.

Body Systems and Functions

CHAPTER 5

Carbs, Fats, Proteins
and
The Faulty Food Pyramid

The Dietary Guidelines for America are incorrect nutritionally. The four basic food groups have been regarded as the cornerstone of a good diet: meat, poultry, and fish; dairy products and eggs; cereals and grains; fruits and vegetables. Throughout our lives the importance of including a balance of each of these groups in our diets has been stressed as a foundation for health. Yet I believe that these principles are upside down and should focus more on the importance of living foods such as vegetables, fruits, and healthy fats.

When we follow the Food Pyramid, our diets contain 75% acid ash foods and only 25% alkaline ash foods. Fruits and vegetables should make up 80% of the diet. Bread, cereal, fish, chicken, and meat affect the acid level of your body, and the acid level of your body affects your health. If the acid ash produced by food is not neutralized, your body will become so toxic that it can no longer function.

To correct the Pyramid, protein should be considered the most important macro nutrient, and complex carbohydrates should be emphasized over simple carbohydrates. In addition, essential fatty acids need to be in proper proportion. More omega-3s and far less omega-6s.

Carbohydrates

Carbohydrates are, or are converted to, sugar. The Dietary Guidelines recommend 45-65% of the diet should be carbohydrates. Carbohydrates are a source of quick energy for the body. There are three types of carbohydrates: simple, complex, and fibrous carbohydrates.

Simple carbohydrates are sugars and are absorbed into the bloodstream rapidly. When digested, carbohydrates are changed by enzymes into a simple sugar form called "glucose". Glucose is one of the building blocks of starches. Glucose, fructose, and galactose inhibit the fat releasing hormone (glucagon) necessary for losing weight.

Chemically, fructose is a hexose that is just the mirror image of glucose (an isomer) that is active. Fruit naturally contains enzymes, vitamins, minerals, and fiber, which help with digestion.

Fruit and milk contain simple sugars and are full of nutrients, but not all simple sugars are healthy. Products containing refined fructose often lack amino acids, vitamins, minerals, and fiber and burden the liver. Fructose promotes disease more readily than glucose because glucose is metabolized by every cell in the body, and fructose must be metabolized by the liver.

Animal studies show that the livers of animals fed large amounts of fructose develop fatty deposits and cirrhosis. This is similar to the livers of alcoholics. These studies show that fructose consumption induces insulin resistance, impaired glucose tolerance, hyperinsulinemia, hypertriglyceridemia, and hypertension in animal models.

The processing of foods changes the molecular structure and exchanges nutrients and taste for economic mass production. Sugar and chemical nutrients are added back in to revive the dead food. These refined sugars do not provide vitamins, minerals, or fiber. They are considered empty calories. A high intake of these sugars is associated with cavities and can contribute to high triglyceride levels and heart disease. High glucose levels are very toxic to the pancreas and kidneys.

One of the worst ways to start off your day is to eat doughnuts for breakfast. They have no nutritional value, given that they are made of trans fats (35-40%), sugar and white flour, and have between 200 to 300 calories.

Every time you drink a can of soda or a glass of orange juice, eat a scoop of fat-free ice cream or honey, eat desserts, breakfast cereals, cookies, cakes, or candy, your pancreas is using up your storage and supply of insulin.

White potatoes convert to glucose, and when they are cooked at high temperatures in trans fat oils (canola, soybean, safflower, and corn), acrylamide is created. Sugar is often added to french fries. It has been noted that one french fry is worse for your health than one cigarette due to the damaging free radicals.

After eating sugar, you typically feel a rush of energy. The sugar levels rise, and the pancreas releases a hormone called insulin. Insulin moves sugar from the blood into the cells, where the sugar can be used as a source of energy. Temporarily, your blood sugar dips, and you crave more simple sugars, which sets up the sugar craving cycle otherwise known as a sugar addiction.

Read the ingredients on food labels, and look for any form of the word sugar: brown sugar, white table sugar, sugar cane, cane syrup, corn syrup, high-fructose corn syrup, glucose syrup, honey, molasses, maple syrup, maltodextrin, fruit juice concentrates, and any ingredients that end in "-ose", like sucrose, glucose, lactose, dextrose, maltose, and fructose.

The food industry is not concerned about your health; they are concerned about sales. They cook away from 4 to 12 essential foods elements, the nutrients. Flavor enhancers (chemicals known as excitotoxins) spike our taste buds and creates more cravings for processed foods. Real foods like broccoli, carrots, celery, and romaine lettuce are tasteless in comparison to chemically-induced flavors. Yet real foods are the only foods that will repair and heal sick body tissues.

Complex carbohydrates are a better choice of energy. They are used immediately or are stored in the liver and muscles for later. While they are also broken down into sugars, these carbohydrates slowly move into the bloodstream and cells, unlike simple carbohydrates that dissipate quickly. They are packed with fiber, vitamins, and minerals.

One serving of grains on the food pyramid, equals one slice of bread, one cup of ready-to-eat cold cereal, or one-half cup of pasta. A restaurant order of linguine is about three cups. A single bagel equals five slices of bread.

Bread should have at least three grams of fiber per serving (whole grain bread has more nutrition). Brown rice, wild rice, muesli, oat bran, oatmeal, buckwheat, barley, and millet have anywhere from 3 to 11g of fiber per serving.

Avoid bread that is bleached, enriched, processed, or refined. Refined flour is made through a process that breaks down the grain and strips it of its nutrients. Whole wheat bread is 100% wheat flour but not necessarily 100% whole grain. 100% whole grain means that the flour has not been refined.

Complex (starchy) and fibrous carbohydrates include brown rice, sweet potatoes, oatmeal, brown pastas, legumes, whole grains, asparagus, broccoli, cauliflower, onions, spinach, peppers and most varieties of dark green leafy vegetables.

Beware of baby carrots. Defective carrots that cannot be sold because of deformities or appearance are shaved-down to form baby carrots. Once the natural protective covering is shaved off, the baby carrots are then preserved by dipping in chlorine, the same chlorine used for your pool. If kept in your refrigerator for a few days, a white covering of chlorine will resurface on the carrots.

Eating complex and fibrous carbohydrates will balance insulin. It will stabilize blood sugar, sharpen concentration, and enhance your mood, resulting in improved physical, mental, and emotional health.

The glycemic index is a measure of how rapidly food will cause your blood sugar to increase. Glucose is used as the reference point for the index, with a rating of 100 on the scale. Table sugar has a rating of 65; a bagel, 72; sweet potatoes, 54; an apple, 36; watermelon, 72. Basically, the higher the rating on the glycemic index, the bigger impact the food will have on your blood sugar level. Fructose is very low glycemic food, yet it is one of the major reasons people are overweight. Apple juice, chocolate, and cherries should not be eaten if your goal is to lose weight.

It is not what we eat that counts, but what we digest and assimilate.

THE GRAINS OF THE BIBLE: BARLEY AND WHEAT

The Promised Land is described as "a land of wheat and barley" (*Deuteronomy 8:8*). Known to improve potency, vigor, and strength, barley has been consumed for thousands of years. Roman gladiators ate barley before their contests for bursts of strength. In *John 6:9-13*, the young boy brought Jesus five barley loaves, with which He fed thousands.

Barley and wheat sprouts, known as cereal grasses, contain four essential compounds largely absent from our diets:

- Antioxidant enzymes
- Chlorophyll
- High-quality vegetable proteins
- Trace minerals

You can juice them yourself at home or consume a green super-food powder containing the dried cereal-grass juices. A variety of super-food powders can be found in health food stores.

FIBER: ANOTHER KIND OF CARBOHYDRATE

Fiber refers to carbohydrates that cannot be digested nor absorbed by the body. It aids in digestion and offers protection against some diseases. It is present in all edible plants including fruits, vegetables, grains and legumes. Fiber is not found in meat.

Studies confirmed that a diet high in fiber reduces the risk of heart disease, diverticulitis, diabetes, and constipation.

Current recommendations are 20-35 grams of fiber per day. You can increase your fiber intake by:

- Replacing white rice, bread, and pasta with whole grain products, and using unrefined, unbleached grains or sprouts such as spelt, brown rice, quinoa, and millet.
- Opting for whole fruits over juices.
- Substituting legumes for meat in chili and soups.
- Starting the morning with a bowl of healthy cereal.

Examples of food with fiber:

Kashi® cereal, 1 cup	10 grams fiber
Lentils, ½ cup	8 grams fiber
Brussels sprouts, 1 cup	6 grams fiber
Potato, 1 large	5 grams fiber
Pear or Apple, 1 medium	4 grams fiber

Fats

Society is buying low fat or non fat foods, and consciously watching fat grams; however, people are getting fatter, not losing weight as one would expect.

To function properly, our bodies require dietary fat. It serves as an energy source. Fat helps our bodies absorb fat-soluble vitamins such as A, D, E, and K. The lower amount of natural oils in our foods are contributing to slowed digestion, constipation (due to lack of lubrication), and hormonal deficiencies and imbalances.

The brain is composed primarily of fat – the right kinds make you smart. If the diet is too high in saturated fat, the wrong kinds of fat, it will reduce your intelligence.

Fat is essentially a storage form of fuel. The body converts excess carbohydrate into fat to be burned later when there is no ready source of carbohydrate. The body can draw upon this fat, which is located all over the body, when the nutritional input from the intestinal tract is insufficient to meet the demand.

Fats pack the highest caloric value into the smallest space so that normal reserves of fuel for muscular activity and the maintenance of body temperature can be most economically stored.

Another type of fat that is entirely abnormal is the accumulation of fat from which the overweight person suffers. This abnormal fat is also a potential reserve of fuel, but unlike the normal reserves, it is not available to the body in a nutritional emergency. It is locked away in a fixed deposit and is not kept in a current account, as are the normal reserves.

When an obese person tries to reduce by starving himself, he will first lose his normal fat reserves. When these are exhausted he begins to burn up structural fat, and only as a last resort will the body yield its abnormal reserves, though by that time the person usually feels so weak and hungry that the diet is abandoned.

Of the three macro nutrients – fats, carbohydrates, and proteins – fats yield the greatest energy per gram. The good news is that, when consuming fats, your body produces less insulin and burns fat stores for fuel. By including fat in your diet, you will feel less hungry and keep your fat-burning furnace running longer.

Most of the fats in your diet should be monounsaturated and omega-3 fats. For the greatest health benefit, a combination of the fats described below should be consumed – each provides a different nutritional component.

Oils can cause aging, clotting, inflammation, cancer, and weight gain. They are polyunsaturated fats and turn rancid when exposed to oxygen.

BEST SOURCES OF DIETARY FAT

Omega-3 Fatty Acids

Found in fatty, cold-water fish (salmon, herring, sardines, and anchovies), walnuts, some seeds (pumpkin seeds, hemp seeds, and flax seeds), and flax seed oil.

The anti-inflammatory properties of omega-3 fatty acids can have a positive impact on, or even prevent, serious degenerative illnesses such as, heart disease, hypertension, rheumatoid arthritis, Alzheimer's, diabetes, and more.

Omega-3 fatty acids are beneficial in preserving heart, breast, and bone health. They are beneficial for depression and help protect against prostate and breast malignancies and some types of dementia.

Monounsaturated Fat

This fat boosts immunity and helps lower blood pressure, blood sugar, and cholesterol levels. Monounsaturated fat is the primary source of fat in the Mediterranean diet.

Good sources of these fats that provide health benefits are extra virgin olive oil, avocado oil, and almond, flax seed, walnut, and macadamia nut oils. They are available at health-food stores.

These nut- and seed-derived oils are usually more expensive than vegetable oils – a 16-ounce bottle of flax seed oil costs about three times what you would pay for the same size bottle of refined soy oil. Because a little goes a long way, not much is needed to add distinctive flavors and variety to cooking.

Extra virgin olive oil is made from the first press of freshly harvested olives. The olives are cold-pressed with a minimum of refining (no heat or chemicals used for extraction). The result is an oil with very low acidity and high levels of phenols, which contain flavonoids – biologically active compounds that are remarkably high in antioxidants.

Unrefined Polyunsaturated Fat

This fat, found in walnut oil and natural vegetable oils that have not been chemically processed, is a source of omega-6 fatty acids. Small doses (no more than one tablespoon daily) are necessary to provide a healthful ratio of omega-6 to omega-3, but they can be harmful when consumed in the high amounts that are typical in the American diet.

Avoid hydrogenated oils, trans fats, and saturated fats. These are found in beef, pork, lamb, chicken, and dairy products, as well as in cookies, crackers, and other processed foods.

EFA (ESSENTIAL FATTY ACID) DEFICIENCY

EFA deficiency is often missed or overlooked by most doctors. Symptoms of EFA deficiency include:

Dry, lifeless hair	High cholesterol
Frequent colds and flu	Lack of endurance
Indigestion, gas, bloating	Lack of motivation
Dry skin	High blood pressure
Immune system disorders	Split nails
Forgetfulness, memory issues	Aching joints
Dry mucus membranes	Depression
Fatigue, poor energy	Arthritis
Cardiovascular disease	Constipation
Chest pain	Breast cancer

COOKING TIPS

Refined "vegetable oils," including corn and soy oils, are best avoided, due to the harmful compounds that are produced in the process of refining.

Do not cook with flax seed oil, borage, or evening primrose oils.

Grape seed oil, extra virgin olive oil, and organic butter can be add after cooking.

Smoke Point

The smoke point of an oil or fat is the temperature at which the heated fat begins to break down, release smoke, and give a burned taste to food.

Oils that have smoke points of about 350°F or higher are good for sauteing and stir-frying. They include almond, macadamia nut, and sesame oils.

Oils with low smoke points – about 225°F – include flax seed oil and unrefined sunflower oil. They are best used raw and/or in baking.

HOW MUCH IS ENOUGH?

All oils contain about 14g of fat, or 126 calories, per tablespoon.

The National Research Council recommends limiting fats to 30% of your daily calorie intake and cholesterol consumption to 30% of that. The emphasis should be on fish, skinless poultry, lean meats, and low-fat or non-fat dairy products, and cutting back on fried and other fatty foods such as pastries, spreads, and dressings.

TRANS FATS

Found in many foods including french fries, fried chicken, doughnuts, cookies, pastries, and crackers, trans fats are artery-clogging fats that are formed when vegetable oils are hardened into margarine or shortening.

Cereals and waffles can also contain trans fats. Read the ingredient label, and look for shortening, hydrogenated oil, or partially hydrogenated oil. The higher up the list these ingredients appear, the more trans fats there are.

Trans fats act like plastic wrap around your cells, keeping toxins in (free radicals) and keeping nutrients and oxygen out.

Corn chips, potato chips, tortilla chips, etc. are also high in trans fat. Some companies are making changes and produce chips without the trans fat; however, they still cook them in high temperatures that will potentially cause the formation of carcinogenic substances like acrylamide.

TRIGLYCERIDES

Triglycerides are chemicals composed primarily of simple fats.

The structure of triglycerides makes it easy for the fats to be stored in food, thus stored in the body and transported in the blood stream.

A high level of triglycerides on a blood test simply means a lot of fat in the blood.

CANOLA OIL

Canola is an acronym for **CAN**ada **O**il **L**ow **A**cid. It was developed in response to a need by the food industry for a cheap alternative to olive oil. "Canola" is *not* a plant. This oil is manufactured from the rapeseed plant, which is in the mustard and cabbage family and considered toxic in large amounts.

By using hexane solvents (a component of gasoline) and other chemicals and heat to strip oil from the rapeseed plant, the oil turns from healthy omega-3s into rancid, smelly trans-fatty acids in higher concentrations than even soybean, corn, cottonseed, and safflower oils. Though it is not listed on the labels, research at the University of Florida at Gainesville revealed that canola and rapeseed oils sold in the USA contained as much as 4.6% trans fat.

In industry, it is used as a lubricant, in the manufacture of biodiesel fuel and soap, in color printing processes, and to make synthetic rubber. Before the canola became popular, rapeseed was mainly grown to produce lubricating products for ships.

The use of canola over time may cause blindness, nervous disorders, clumping of blood cells and depression of the immune system, anemia, constipation, increased incidence of heart disease and cancer, low birth weights in infants, and irritability. Many of these have not appeared in medical journals, and long-term research has not been done to substantiate or refute the claims.

Animal studies have linked canola oil with reduced platelet count, shorter life span, and increased need for vitamin E. In 1985, the Federal Register (official journal of the federal government of the United States) stated that the FDA outlawed canola oil in infant formulas because it retarded growth.

If you want to research this further, go to the internet. I used a variety of resources to make my conclusions. Although there is a very informative video on YouTube, "How It's Made – Canola Oil", it inaccurately refers to rapeseed plant as the "Canola plant". I stopped using Canola before my research. Now I think I will use it to polish furniture – it leaves a nice shine!

<u>BUTTER</u>

Butter is slightly higher in saturated fats than margarine – 8g per tablespoon compared to 5g – but has greater nutritional benefits. Butter also enhances the absorption of many other nutrients in foods, it tastes better, it can enhance the flavors of foods, and it has been around for centuries.

High quality butter has a beneficial effect on the immune system. But fats have twice the calories per unit measure as sugar, so keep that in mind if you are counting calories.

MARGARINE

All margarines are made from assorted vegetable oils that have been heated to extremely high temperatures. This means that the oils will become rancid. After that, a nickel catalyst is added along with hydrogen atoms to solidify it. Nickel is a toxic heavy metal and trace amounts always remain in the finished product. Finally, deodorants and colorings are added to remove margarine's horrible smell (from the rancid oils) and unappetizing gray color. In the solidification process, harmful trans-fatty acids are created, which are carcinogenic and mutagenic.

Facts about margarine:

- Increases heart disease in women by 53% over eating the same amount of butter, found a Harvard medical study
- Is very high in trans-fatty acids
- Has been around for less than 100 years
- Has few benefits, and those have been added!
- Increases the risk of cancer by up to five fold and triples the risk of coronary heart disease
- Increases total cholesterol and LDL (the bad cholesterol) and lowers HDL cholesterol (the good cholesterol)
- Lowers quality of breast milk
- Decreases immune and insulin responses
- Margarine is only one molecule away from being plastic

Purchase a tub of margarine, and leave it in your garage or shaded area. Within a couple of days you will note a couple of things: No flies – not even those pesky fruit flies will go near it (that should tell you something). It does not rot or smell different. Nothing will grow on it – not even microorganisms – because it is nearly plastic. Would you melt Tupperware® and spread it on your toast?

COCONUT OIL

Part of the confusion about coconut oil relates to its content of saturated fat that is burned for energy rather than stored as body fat. Fresh coconut juice is one of the highest sources of electrolytes known to man, and can be used to prevent dehydration. Some remote areas of the world even use coconut juice intravenously, short-term, to help hydrate critically ill patients and in emergency situations.

100% raw, unrefined coconut oil from Kerala, India is not refined, bleached, deodorized, or hydrogenated (which damages the oil and makes it toxic). It helps to naturally increase metabolism as much as 25% – great for those with weight and thyroid concerns. It burns fat, increases energy, and boosts thyroid and immune systems. Unsaturated fats such as corn and safflower oils can decrease thyroid efficiency and lower metabolic rates. Coconut oil from Kerala, India does not contain dangerous trans fats that are found in unsaturated vegetable oils, margarine, shortening, etc.

Benefits of coconut oil from Kerala, India:

- One third fewer calories per gram
- Easily digestible

- Quick energy source for cells
- Anti-microbial properties
- No trans fat
- Cooking with it does not create free radicals

IS SATURATED FAT BAD?

Certain saturated fats are necessary to human health (your brain is comprised mostly of saturated fat). Saturated fats are not the primary perpetrator of weight gain – they come in three classes, of which the medium-chain type can actually help to increase metabolism and burn fat. (The real culprits in weight gain are refined grains and sugars.)

Coconut oil contains naturally-occurring saturated fat. Mary Enig, an internationally known expert in fats and lipid biochemistry and author of the well-researched "fat information bible", Know Your Fats, promotes coconut oil and its ability to boost the immune system and keep the body in good health.

SUMMARY

1. Why you need fat:

- A layer of protection for the abdominal organs
- Keeps you warm
- Acts as fuel – 9 calories of energy per gram consumed
- Absorbs and transports oil soluble nutrients like vitamins A, D, E, and K (A and E are strong anti-cancer agents)
- Regulates hormones
- Needed for cellular reproduction

2. Types of fats:

- Saturated fats come from animal sources
  - Associated with increasing cholesterol
  - Difficult to break down
- Unsaturated fats
  - Help carry excess hydrogen from the body
  - Break down easier, keep the blood vessel walls clean and plaque free
  - Most desirable to consume
- Hydrogenated fat
  - Hydrogenation process – heated to 248-410°F and combined with hydrogen – makes it hard to digest.
  - Excess hydrogen stiffens joints and deactivates some digestive enzymes
  - Need to avoid

3. Essential Fatty Acids (EFAs)

- Omega-3
  - Cold water fish, fish oils, flax seeds
  - Known for blood thinning effect
  - Decrease high blood pressure and carry oxygen through the body, blood, and brain.
- Omega-6
  - Thicken the blood
  - Most common fat and is usually overeaten

- Omega-9
  - Created from omega-3 and omega-6 (should be 1:1 ratio for proper production)
- Best EFA supplemental sources: Borage, evening primrose, cod liver, fish, flax seed, hemp, and krill oils.

OIL PULLING

This method pulls disease elements out of the body system and restores health. You can do this two more times during the day if you want to detox faster. Make sure you do it on an empty stomach, however.

Using sunflower oil, take one tablespoon of oil first thing in the morning before breakfast. Do not swallow it.

For 15 to 20 minutes, slowly wash and suck the oil inside the mouth, pulling it through the teeth with closed mouth. Really move your chin and chew so that a lot of saliva is drawn; that means mouth digestion. The oil is viscous, but the longer it is in your mouth, the thinner it becomes.

The oil should not be swallowed because it has become toxic. Poisons are drawn from the blood through the mucous membrane of the mouth, and the discarded oil contains large amounts of bacteria and harmful material. If we would look at a drop of this liquid through a microscope, we would see all kind of moving fibers – those are microbes in the first stage of their growth.

Spit it out in the toilet when your mouth is full, and rinse your mouth out well. The oil will have turned white like wool. (If the liquid is still yellow, you did not work with the oil long enough.)

After spitting out the oil, the mouth has to be washed intensely with water several times. Rinse your mouth with ½ tsp baking soda, ½ tsp sea salt in 4 oz warm water. Brush your teeth.

Drink two or three 8 oz glasses of water after this procedure.

Reported Cures with Oil Pulling

Mouth and gum disease, stiff joints, allergies, asthma, diabetes and high blood sugar, constipation, migraines, bronchitis, eczema, heart disease, kidney disease, lung disease, leukemia, arthritis, meningitis, insomnia, menopause and other hormonal issues, cancer, AIDS, chronic infections, varicose veins, high blood pressure, polio, cracked heels.

The first sign of improvement is in the teeth – they will become firm and white. Other healing indications: fresh, relaxed feeling on waking up, disappearing dark pouches below the eyes, renewed appetite and energy, better memory, and deeper sleep.

The tongue is mapped by organ-locations — that is, different sections of the tongue are connected to meridians associated with the kidneys, lungs, spleen, liver, heart, pancreas, small intestines, stomach, colon, and spine. Thus, an oil mouth-massage soothes and stimulates the key meridians where taste meets organ.

Proteins

Protein is crucial in balancing hormones and responsible for antibody production in the immune system. It builds and repairs muscle and is essential for skin health and wound healing.

Protein is broken down through digestion into amino acids, building blocks considered to be mood enhancers, helping to control depression and anxiety. It is also warming to the body.

The best sources of protein will contain all 8 essential amino acids, which come from the diet. Foods like meats, fish, poultry, and eggs should be certified organic or free range since the use of antibiotics and hormones, used to make the animals grow faster, are detrimental for human consumption.

Brown rice, nuts, seeds, and wheat are high in protein but are missing one or more of the essential amino acids. When brown rice is combined with beans in the diet, it is considered a complete protein. Wheat bread combined with nut butters, seeds, nuts, or legumes, along with salads, will also provide a more complete source of protein.

Protein needs vary according to the ability to digest and utilize it. Some nutritionists suggest that women need 35-45g and men, 45-55g daily. Yet others suggest that 25g per day is sufficient.

Protein causes an acid condition in the body. The more protein you eat than what the body can handle, especially animal protein, the more it places your body into a state of catabolism.

Catabolism is the process of rapid burning of excess protein, giving a false sense of strength.

Catabolism produces uric acid, which irritates the body, especially the nervous system. The body then makes an effort to protect itself by stealing calcium and other alkalizing minerals such as magnesium, sodium, and potassium from bones and teeth in order to buffer the uric acid, leaving the body overstimulated and calcium depleted. This combination causes premature aging.

The kidneys are also stressed because they work to strip the nitrogen from the excess protein in the blood stream. Problems like weak kidneys, kidney stones, or gout may manifest.

PROTEIN BREAKDOWN

Drinking fluids with meals, especially cold drinks, interferes with the production of hydrochloric acid, which is needed to create the proper pH in the stomach for pepsin (a digestive enzyme) to break down the protein into amino acids. It is essential to have the proper pH in the gut as well as the correct concentration of stomach juices.

CHOOSING CLEAN MEATS

Dishes made from pork come from an unclean animal. Clean animals that chew their cud, like cows and deer, have an advanced digestive system that includes an alimentary canal and a secondary cud receptacle. They have three stomachs to process and refine their clean, vegetation-based food in a process that can take up to twenty-four hours.

Pigs do not limit their diet to vegetation. They will eat anything they can find, including their own young and sick or dead pigs from the same pen. Therefore, pork contains poisons and by-products that can harm you, including the destructive enzymes cadaverine and putrescine.

The Bible's guidelines: Choose meat from animals that have cloven hooves *and* chew their cud. There are no exceptions to this rule. If an animal has only one of these qualities, its meat is unclean according to this rule.

One of the most recent treatments on food is irradiation. Gamma rays from radioactive isotopes are used to kill parasites and insects, slow ripening, or dehydrate. Irradiation lengthens the unrefrigerated shelf life of foods and slows the maturing process of fruits and vegetables so they look better longer. In the US, only a limited variety of food – including fresh pork – may legally be irradiated. Irradiation works by the "formation of electrically charged, highly reactive molecules that damage living cells."

TOXINS IN MEAT

Beef fat is marbled throughout the product. If beef cattle are injected with female hormones, growth hormones, steroids, and antibiotics, these toxins are stored in their fat.

"If we eat the flesh of animals, we are but eating chewed and digested grasses. If we drink milk or eat butter, it is the same thing; namely, chewed grass, only that in such cases, we get the vital, or life, principle secondhand because much of the life has been used by the animal whose flesh we eat. But whenever you cut through the flesh of any animal, you have as much venous blood as arterial blood. The venous blood contains the waste matter and debris of that animal's cells. That animal flesh is subject to putrefaction and produces very poisonous alkaloids, while vegetables in the process of decay do not produce alkaloids or putrefaction." *Advanced Treatise in Herbology, Edward Shook, p. 101*

POSITIVE PROTEIN SOURCES

A cup of cooked broccoli contains 40 calories, but it contains over four grams of protein. It contains more than one gram of protein for every ten calories.

One cup rice and one half cup of beans will supply about 178 calories and 6.4g protein. That is 28 calories for each gram of protein – a very favorable ratio and one reason that this combination is one of the world's most common sources of both energy and protein.

Leafy greens are surprisingly high in protein, with one cup of mustard greens containing 16 calories and 1.7g of protein – a 10 to 1 ratio.

Vegetarian diets can be nutritious if "calories only" foods such as sugars, refined starches, fats and oils, and alcohol are avoided in favor of protein-rich foods.

NEGATIVE PROTEIN SOURCES

A piece of fudge has 150 calories for every gram of protein.

A tablespoon of jam has essentially no protein for its 50 calories.

Hundreds of calories are taken in every day with absolutely no protein. This nutrient debt of protein destroys the balance. If this is done too often in a day, the balance will never be restored. In an effort to get the amount of protein needed, concentrated protein foods like cheese, eggs, or meat would be required (highly acidic foods).

PROTEIN FROM TURKEY

Turkey is high in nutrients, low in saturated fat and calories, and supplies lots of amino acids. The skinless breast of turkey is one of the leanest-meat protein sources. Three ounces provide about 26g of protein, contains B vitamins, zinc, and selenium, and is a good source of niacin, and vitamins B_6 and B_{12}.

BEANS

Beans are full of complex carbohydrates, which give us energy. They are very low in fat and an excellent source of soluble fiber, which can lower blood sugar. Eating 50g of fiber per day has the potential to lower blood sugar by as much as 10%!

Fiber in beans is a source of roughage. However, many people avoid eating beans because of embarrassing gas, caused by carbohydrates in the beans that cannot be broken down into simpler sugars and digested. These undigested sugars become food for the bacteria that resides in the gut. Bacteria metabolize sugars in a fermentation process.

To help reduce gas, soak beans overnight, discard the soaking water, and cover with fresh water. Bring to a boil, then drain, and rinse again. This removes some of the offending sugars, thereby reducing the gas-producing potential. The beans are ready for cooking.

COW'S MILK

Milk and cheese are high in protein and low in carbohydrates. The problem is that cow's milk is suited for larger, heavier bones. Consider the cow – it also has a much larger liver in proportion to its body than the human, especially a human baby. A study from the University of Liverpool warns: "Milk is for baby cows, not for baby humans" - or adult humans, for that matter.

Commercially available cow's milk is pasteurized and homogenized (for easier digestion), which kills harmful bacteria and destroys many of the natural enzymes. Louis Pasteur's process (which was originally designed to prevent beer spoilage) has been in widespread use for a little more than a century, though non-pasteurized milk is not hazardous. It's just a lot tougher to regulate it and make money from it.

By legislating against the sale or distribution of raw milk, states force farmers to sell their milk (at a fraction of market value) to the big milk processors. This creates a paper trail on the milk, which can be used as the basis for collecting tax revenue from the processors and the farmers.

Cow's milk has been linked to health concerns including prostate problems and (ironically) bone fractures. And dairy causes mucus to form in the lungs and throat. Think about how your body responds to milk when you have a cold. The stomach creates a lining of mucus to envelope pathogens. So if milk creates mucus when you are not sick, and even more when you are sick, what conclusions can you draw?

Raw milk is healthier, better for you, and tastes better, too, and raw milk drinkers enjoy increased resistance to colds and flu, weight loss, and relief from arthritis pain.

Goat's milk is founded on experience that goes back thousands of years – ask a person who raises goats about the health supporting benefits. Goat's milk compares favorably to mother's milk and is more easily assimilated than cow's milk because the fat globules in goat's milk are five times smaller than those in cow's milk, making it easier on the liver and aiding in the digestive processes. Goat's milk also has more alkaline properties than the cow's milk.

Nut milks are also good alternatives. However, soy will pump you full of estrogen-mimicking compounds, which can depress your thyroid and make you put on weight. It also contains an acid that blocks the absorption of calcium.

CHAPTER 6

Diets
and
Body Mass Index

The Body Mass Index (BMI) measures your weight relative to your height and is calculated as your weight, in kilograms, divided by your height, in centimeters, squared. The guidelines for determining risk factors associated with obesity are: BMI below 18.5 is underweight, between 18.5 and 24.9 is normal, between 25.0 and 29.9 is overweight, and 30.0 and over is obese.

Three tips to reduce body mass index:

1. Get active. Exercise for one half hour daily, and you will lose 5-7% of your body weight per year.

2. Cut out white breads and sugars. Substitute whole grains for refined flours and sugars, and you will automatically reduce the number of calories that you consume daily.

3. Eat more fresh vegetables. Fresh vegetables, especially raw, are a significant source of many of the vitamins and minerals that your body needs daily. They are high in nutrition and low in calories.

Diets

THE ATKINS DIET

The Atkins diet book sold 15 million copies in the US. It was on the New York Times bestseller list for four years. The original Atkins diet promoted eating unlimited amounts of beef, sausage, butter, and cheese. This diet may be good for short-term weight loss, but it is not great for optimal health.

Atkins Diet Pitfalls:

- Stresses low carbohydrates
- Allows two-thirds of calories from animal fat
- Does not work for everyone
- One third of the population require a high-carb diet
- Ketosis occurs if you do not have enough carbohydrates to burn as fuel. Ketones are the breakdown product as your body uses fat. This is not a healthy condition to intentionally induce and leaves a strange breath odor.
- Must count carbs – cumbersome and time-consuming
- Recommends sucralose (Splenda®) - health risks
- Encourages you to eat nuts, which have health benefits but are high in omega-6s.
- Not enough exercise – only 30 min/day, but you need 60 min/day to lose weight
- Food quality is as important as the type of food you eat
- Allows processed meats such as bacon, and low-carb energy bars

To improve the Atkins diet:

- Meats – should come from grass-fed livestock
- Milk – give consideration for lactose intolerance
- Fish – avoid types of fish which contain mercury and PCBs

Low-carb diets promote short-term weight loss. Healthy eating is not quite as simple (or boring) as living on fat and protein. You can have carbohydrates, but you must know how to choose them. Dr. Atkins passed away in 2003 at age 72. He was 6' 0" and 258 lbs.

THE ZONE DIET

This diet is about maintaining hormones generated by the food you eat within controlled insulin zones. To stay within the Zone, you need to eat 40% carbs, 30% low fat protein, and 30% mono-unsaturated fats and drink lots of water.

THE BLOOD TYPE DIET ("Eat Right For Your Type" by Peter D'Adamo)

This book is about 64% accurate, but it is still worth reading.

FOOD COMBINING

Properly combining foods promotes better digestion, increased energy, weight loss, better elimination, less feeling of hunger, better nutrient absorption, and a sense of well-being. Wrong combinations of foods, however, can cause gas, indigestion, weight gain, and other problems.

Food Combining Guidelines:

- Eat proteins with vegetables.
- Eat starches with vegetables and other starches.
- Eat protein foods and starches at separate meals.
- Eat fats and proteins at separate meals.
- Eat fruits alone.
- Eat melons alone, or leave them alone!
- Avoid eating carbohydrates (pastas & potatoes) in evening meal. They digest quickly and turn into glucose. If you are not active after dinner, the glucose goes directly to your fat cells.

THE CHEW, CHEW DIET

Drink your solids, chew your liquids, and chew each bite 25-50 times.

THE DANIEL FAST

Background

Daniel and his three friends had been deported to Babylon when Nebuchadnezzar and the Babylonians had conquered Judah (2 Kings 24:13-14). Daniel and his three friends were put into the Babylonian court servant training program. Part of the program was learning Babylonian customs, beliefs, laws, and practices. The eating habits of the Babylonians were not in complete agreement with the Mosaic law. As a result, Daniel asked if he and his three friends could be excused from eating the meat (which was likely sacrificed to Babylonian false gods and idols).

"In those days I, Daniel, was mourning three full weeks. I ate no pleasant food, no meat or wine came into my mouth, nor did I anoint myself at all, till three whole weeks were fulfilled." *Daniel 10:2-3 NKJV*

Fasting is between you and God. Do not compare your sacrifice to others. Seek God to lead you. Pray for wisdom. God honors your sacrifice. He will be honored, and you will be blessed.

Fasting is always tied to prayer. Fasting alone, without intimate time spent in prayer, reading, and studying the Bible, is just a diet. If you focus only on what you can and cannot eat, you will lose sight of the purpose of the fast. Increase your devotional time with prayer and Bible reading, and you will find added strength and comfort through the scriptures and through your prayer time with the Lord.

A Daniel fast is observed by many of the church body during the beginning of each year. This is powerfully significant when there is unity with other believers. You are giving your first fruits to Him.

Foods included in the Daniel Fast

You are not limited to any specific amount of food but rather to the kinds of food that you can eat. The Daniel Fast is limited to fruits, vegetables, and water. Abstention from meat products for a certain amount of time is also required.

On the Daniel fast, you are allowed to eat:

- All fruits – These can be fresh, frozen, dried, juiced, or canned. Fruits include, but are not limited to: apples, apricots, bananas, blackberries, blueberries, boysenberries, cantaloupe, cherries, cranberries, figs, grapefruit, grapes, guava, honeydew melon, kiwi, lemons, limes, mangoes, nectarines, oranges, papayas, peaches, pears, pineapples, plums, prunes, raisins, raspberries, strawberries, tangelos, tangerines, and watermelon.

- All vegetables – These can be fresh, frozen, dried, juiced, or canned. Vegetables include, but are not limited to: artichokes, asparagus, beets, broccoli, brussels sprouts, cabbage, carrots, cauliflower, celery, chili peppers, collard greens, corn, cucumbers, eggplant, garlic, ginger root, kale, leeks, lettuce, mushrooms, mustard greens, okra, onions, parsley, potatoes, radishes, rutabagas, scallions, spinach, sprouts, squashes, sweet potatoes, tomatoes, turnips, watercress, yams, and zucchini.

- Veggie burgers are also an option as long as you are not allergic to soy.

- All whole grains – Including, but not limited to: whole wheat, brown rice, millet, quinoa, oats, barley, grits, whole wheat pasta, whole wheat tortillas, rice cakes, and popcorn.

- All nuts and seeds – Including, but not limited to: sunflower seeds, cashews, peanuts, and sesame. Also nut butters including peanut butter.

- All legumes – These can be canned or dried and include, but are not limited to: pinto beans, split peas, lentils, black eyed peas, kidney beans, black beans, cannelloni beans, and white beans.

- All quality oils – Including, but not limited to: olive, grape seed, and sesame oils.

- Beverages – Spring water, distilled water, or other pure types of water.

- Other – Tofu, soy products, vinegar, seasonings, salt, herbs, and spices.

On the Daniel fast, you are *not* allowed to eat:

- All meat and animal products including, but not limited to: beef, lamb, pork, poultry, and fish.

- All dairy products including, but not limited to: milk, cheese, cream, butter, and eggs.

- All sweeteners including, but not limited to: white sugar, raw sugar, honey, syrups, molasses, and cane juice.

- All leavened bread (including Ezekiel Bread, which contains yeast and honey) and baked goods.

- All refined and processed food products including, but not limited to: artificial flavorings, food additives, chemicals, white rice, white flour, and foods that contain artificial preservatives.

- All deep fried foods including, but not limited to: potato chips, French fries, and corn chips.

- All solid fats including shortening, margarine, and lard, as well as any foods that are high in fat.

- Beverages including, but not limited to: coffee, tea, herbal teas, carbonated beverages, energy drinks, and alcohol.

Special Note: If you have health issues, be sure to contact your health professional for advice before committing to any fast including the Daniel fast.

THE RAW FOOD DIET

The premise behind the raw food lifestyle is that heating food above 116°F destroys important living enzymes and other nutrients. By preserving the living elements of food, degenerative disease is prevented, aging is slowed, energy enhanced, and emotional well-being is boosted.

To be considered a raw-foodist, you only need to consume 75% raw food. In a nutshell, you eat nothing cooked – no pasta, no rice and beans, no steamed broccoli, no tofu (made from cooked soybeans). Many raw-foodists are strictly 100% raw and aim for a high percentage of organic food.

To get an almost cooked feeling, purchase a dehydrator. In this way, you can concentrate the flavor and alter the texture of food without heat. Soak nuts (to activate enzymes and calm down enzyme inhibitors), sprout grains (to make them digestible), ferment cabbage, and juice vegetables (you can consume more and feel fuller).

You will feel clean and energized. Also, avoid high fat foods such as macadamia nuts, cashews, and coconut butter if you are counting calories.

THE VEGETARIAN DIET

Vegetarians tend to have a lower risk of heart disease, high blood pressure, type 2 diabetes, and some forms of cancer than non-vegetarians. The American Institute for Cancer Research and the World Cancer Research Fund recommend eating a mainly plant-based diet containing no more than 18 ounces (6 servings) of cooked red meat (beef, pork, and lamb) per week. They also recommend eliminating processed meats such as bacon, ham, sausage, and lunch meat completely.

If you plan to transition to vegetarianism, eat vegetarian the majority of the time but include small amounts of meat, poultry, or fish at first. Some vegetarians include dairy products and eggs, but some (vegans) exclude these. It is possible to eat an unhealthy vegetarian diet that contains too much fat, too many calories, and too little fiber or other nutrients. Plan carefully.

Here are some tips to follow that will help you to get the nutrients that your body needs on a vegetarian diet:

- To calculate how much protein you need in your diet, aim for 0.8-1.2g of protein per kg of your body weight. Rather than trying to improve protein supplementation from amino acids, vegans should eat a variety of plant foods such as whole grain cereals, nuts, seeds, grains, and legumes, and choose whole-grain breads, cereals, rice, and pasta instead of refined products.

- Vitamin B_{12} deficiency may be a problem for those not eating dairy products and eggs, in which case it is important to include vitamin B_{12}-fortified foods such as soy milk, cereals, and meat analogs such as veggie burgers.

- If you eat dairy products, choose calcium-fortified products like a nut milk. Naturally rich sources of calcium are canned salmon or sardines with bones, dark leafy greens, and broccoli.

- To help meet iron needs, choose plant sources of iron-rich foods including legumes (beans), dark green leafy vegetables, dried fruits, seeds, nuts, and iron-fortified cereals. Including foods high in vitamin C with high iron foods helps to improve absorption of iron. These include citrus fruits, broccoli, tomatoes, and green peppers.

- Limit your empty intake of calorie foods such as sweets, sodas, chips, and candy.

Diets and Body Mass Index

CHAPTER 7

The Healing Process
(Putting it all Together)

"This service that you perform is not only supplying the needs of God's people but is also overflowing in many expressions of thanks to God. Because of the service by which you have proved yourselves, men will praise God for the obedience that accompanies your confession of the gospel of Christ, and for your generosity in sharing with them and with everyone else. And in their prayers for you their hearts will go out to you, because of the surpassing grace God has given you. Thanks be to God for his indescribable gift!" *II Cor. 9:12-15 NIV*

"Dear friend, I pray that you may enjoy good health and that all may go well with you, even as your soul is getting along well." *3 John 1:2 NIV*

"Say to him: 'Long life to you! Good health to you and your household! And good health to all that is yours!'" *1 Samuel 25:6 NIV*

"Don't you know that you yourselves are God's temple and that God's Spirit lives in you? If anyone destroys God's temple, God will destroy him; for God's temple is sacred, and you are that temple." *I Cor. 3: 16-17 ESV*

Healing Crisis

When diet and lifestyles change, many people experience an allergic response to the toxic by-products produced when the body's pH is changed for the better. This is called a Herxheimer reaction. It happens as large numbers of dangerous bacteria and yeast organisms die and leave the body.

The key in reversing the body from acid to alkaline is to take the gradual detox approach. You won't feel very well during this time, but your body is responding positively. After this initial detoxification period, you should see significant improvement of your symptoms.

Remember that rapid changes *are* possible. Your health *will* improve quickly. But you *will* feel worse in the process. You may experience unpleasant symptoms such as lack of energy, diarrhea, headaches, or a general feeling of "the blues".

Your conclusion: "I'm miserable." But your body needs time to adjust to processing new foods and attempts to clear obstructions that clog the system. Disease symptoms may manifest as the body makes an effort to remove excess waste through one or more channels of elimination: bowels, skin, kidneys, liver, female reproductive system, or respiratory tract.

When the body tries to remove toxins through these channels the results can include:

- Bowels – nausea, vomiting, diarrhea
- Kidneys – frequent and burning urination, kidney stones
- Skin – rash, pimples, hives, acne, dandruff, itching, body odor
- Liver: headaches, stiffness, irritability, flu
- Respiratory tract: foul breath, runny nose, watery eyes, sneezing, post-nasal drip, earache, sore throat, congestion
- Female reproductive system: PMS, cramps, bloating, irritability, vaginitis

PMS RELIEF

Getting relief may be as simple as taking 1½ tablespoons of cod liver oil daily and eating more fish, grass-fed free-range beef, free-range poultry, walnuts, and flax seed (all of which help boost omega-3 fatty acid levels). Cramps should subside and disappear altogether within three to four months as omega-3 levels rise above that of omega-6s (omega-6 fatty acids promote cramping and cause inflammation).

At that point, you can discontinue the cod liver oil as long as you keep your diet rich in omega-3 foods. Work on eliminating as many foods as possible from your diet that contain omega-6 oils. This can be difficult since most snack foods and bakery products are rich in omega-6 fatty acids.

AM I SICK – OR DETOXING?

Germs are microorganisms, viruses, bacteria, and other life forms that can play a part in disease. Bacteria that resides in the human body is viewed by traditional medicine as something bad that must be destroyed. But germs are not the cause of illness, and killing them off is not the solution.

Germs seek an environment that offers the best opportunity for their sustained existence and propagation. Damaged cells serve as a host, providing nutrition and an accommodating environment for them to thrive. And we are constantly exposed to germs (each of us carries an estimated 100 trillion bacteria both in and on our bodies), so if germs were the cause of disease, we would all be sick all the time.

The wrong kind of food, excessive fatigue, high-intensity events of an accident, long-term or non-stop abuse, or a destructive lifestyle disrupt the normal function of the whole body as well as individual cells. And our cells are susceptible to invaders when vitality and resistance are reduced. Then germs affect our health. They do not attack normal, vital, healthy cells, or tissue and cannot feed on healthy cells.

We live or die at the cellular level. Health, vitality, and resistance to disease is determined by the health of the cells. Cells that are not completely healthy are unable to ward off attack, resistance goes down, germs multiply, and health is impaired.

Pathogenic germs are scavengers to attack damaged cells, which serve as nutrition for them. Germs that invade the inner workings of the body force the body to respond. The responses are unpleasant and signal that the defenses are down.

The body will do all it can to maintain a steady state of homeostasis. A cold, fever, runny nose, and tears are an indication that the body still has enough vitality to defend itself. Toxins are released, and microorganisms (germs) are carrying out their function as scavengers to attack the damage.

"Disease preys on an undernourished body."
 – *Dr. W. Albrecht, Department of Agriculture, University of Missouri*

HELPING THE DETOXIFICATION PROCESS

Methods of assisting the body in cleansing:

- Open the bowels through herbs, enemas, and dietary changes

- Use herbs to add expulsion of mucus: teas, poultices, and essential oils

- Improve elimination through the skin: exercise, sweat baths, skin brushing, and herbs

- Strengthen the kidneys: drink water

Herring's Law of Cure

"The body heals from the top down, the inside out, and in reverse order of symptoms."

- Top down – change attitude about nutrition and supplements. Healing has to start in the mind.

- Inside out – strengthen the body to push out irritants and get rid of toxins.

- In reverse order – you will experience the symptoms that were previously suppressed.

"A discharge that is dormant in the body may again become active, and... you... may become alarmed, but when nature is cleaning house, she stirs up latent, encapsulated conditions that will gradually eliminate. Cleansing, nature is breaking down the stored-up toxic material that has developed in the body from the use of drugs, vaccines, injections, and generally bad living habits. Those who do not understand nature's way of ridding the body of toxins through a discharge, do not understand that when a drug is given to suppress this discharge they are interfering with nature's way of ridding the body of toxic waste. This elimination of toxins by the body is referred to as 'the healing crisis'." *The Science and Practice of Iridology, Bernard Jensen p.164*

"No discipline seems pleasant at the time, but painful. Later on, however, it produces a harvest of righteousness and peace for those who have been trained by it." *Hebrews 12:11 NIV*

"While most patients are looking for a good doctor, the real doctor wants patients who are desirous of learning to live healthfully." *Dr. Bernard Jensen*

Making Gradual Changes

DIET & NUTRITION

The first step is to change sweeteners, from refined sugar to raw sugar, raw honey, natural maple sugar, molasses, sorghum, or date sugar. Sweet cravings can also be satisfied with fresh or dried fruit. Although fruit juices have a very high glycemic index (causing blood sugar to spike), you should begin to replace carbonated beverages with apple, grape, pineapple juices, etc. A very large intake of even natural sweets is still not desirable, however.

Second, refined white flour should be omitted and replaced with less refined flour – more nutritious, earthier, and richer in flavor.

The third major change in diet would be replacing refined vegetable oils, shortening, and margarine with butterfat. A word of caution on excessive amounts, though. A maximum of two tablespoons of butter or ghee (clarified butter) per day is recommended. If butter is not available, sesame oil is probably the lease detrimental vegetable oil and should be used in very small quantities.

Besides foods that contain white flour, white sugar, and refined vegetables oils, others such as most canned, frozen, ready-prepared convenience foods and processed preparations like cheese spreads and hydrogenated peanut butter are best avoided altogether. Those that contain artificial preservatives as well as excessive amounts of sugar and salt also belong in this group. Many fruit juices, dried fruits, nuts, cheeses, frozen vegetables, and even some so-called health foods fall into this category, too.

Please make sure to read the label when purchasing packaged, canned, or bottled foods. Claims such as "enriched" and "fortified" indicates that additives are necessary because the product is not in its natural state. They should also be free of sugar and chemicals.

Shop on the outer perimeter of the store, the produce counter, the dairy section, and the shelves that hold dried beans, peas, rice, and whole grain flours.

The golden rule: purchase foods that are as fresh as possible. These have the highest level of nutrients, especially if they are grown in rich, organic soil. The freshest foods are those that are hand picked from your own garden just before the meal. The next best are those purchased daily from the local vegetable stand or farmer's market.

GUIDELINES

First: Increase the amount of cooked vegetables that you eat every day.

Second: Reduce the amount of protein foods that you eat each day. Serve smaller portions of beef, poultry, and fish, and add more cooked vegetables.

Third: Cook your vegetables less, and include one serving of raw vegetables or fruit every day.

Fourth: Begin to reduce your intake of salt, coffee, tea, cola drinks, and processed snack foods.

Aim for:

- 45% cooked fruits and vegetables
- 30% raw fruits and vegetables
- 25% grains, nuts, seeds, meat, fish, or poultry

If you have been living on a diet of meats, fast foods, processed or prepared ready-made foods, refined carbohydrates, and stimulants such as coffee, tea, cola, or alcoholic drinks, and your body has suffered from this abuse for many years, you may need to extend each phase. How your body responds is the best gauge of how quickly you can change and improve your diet.

And if you have already been following a healthy diet that includes fresh, whole foods such as vegetables and fruits, you may be able to ramp up the timetable to improving your health.

SAMPLE TIMETABLE

Begin: Add whole foods and cooked vegetables.

After 3 or 4 days: Add a serving of fruit.

After 2 weeks: Have one meal a day of only fruit and cooked vegetables. Begin decreasing the amount of health inhibitors you consume (coffee, tea, cola).

After 3 weeks: Begin reducing salt. Increase the amount of cooked vegetables and raw fruits.

After 1 month: Begin reducing the amount of high protein foods. Reduce your intake of one health inhibitor each week (alcohol, cigarettes, chocolate, etc.) and add some lightly cooked or raw vegetables.

Ongoing: Increase the amount of whole foods – fresh fruits and vegetables, and decrease the amount of carbohydrates, cookies, candies, cakes, ice cream, and sodas.

Those who have been slaves to their taste buds rather than listening to the body requirements will find that slow, steady movement toward better health is realistic. You can expect your health to improve within six months to a year without ever considering any radical changes.

The Healing Process (Putting it all Together)

CHAPTER 8

Herbs or Drugs?

Herbs

Definition: "A non-woody plant that dies back to the ground after each growing season; any of various plants (often aromatic) used for medicine or seasoning."

An herbalist or botanic physician is one whose therapeutics are confined to the use of herbs, roots, barks, seeds, flowers, and berries.

"Let your food be your medicine and your medicine be your food."
Hippocrates

"Then God said, "I give you every seed-bearing plant on the face of the whole earth and every tree that has fruit with seed in it. They will be yours for food." *Genesis 1:29 NIV*

As you know, foods influence the structure and function of the human body. Herbs are natural food medicines that alter the structure and function of the body favorably. Foods are not considered drugs unless they are sold for curing, preventing or treating disease. If this provision were not the law, then all foods would be drugs since all foods affect the structure or function of the body.

Herbs are useful when taking a holistic approach to healing - working with the entire body, mind, and spirit and recognizing that all healing is ultimately performed by the body, not by a physician. Choose your herbs by sight, smell, and taste.

Drugs

Definition:

- A substance used as medicine in the treatment of disease

- A narcotic, especially one that is addictive

- In the United States, the legal definition of a drug is anything that affects the structure or function of the body and is sold for the cure, prevention, treatment, or mitigation of a disease.

- Drugs are concentrates, fractionates, and synthetics.

- Many times they are originally made from plants but are altered so the active principle is   isolated   and removed to improve on nature by forcing the body to do something or by numbing. This is not natural, nor is it healthy.

Congress passed the Food and Drug Act in 1906. The responsibility of implementing and enforcing the law was assigned to a division of the Department of Agriculture, the Bureau of Chemistry. This regulatory agency was originally formed in response to food and drug scandals to help protect people.

The name, Bureau of Chemistry, was eventually changed to the Food and Drug Administration (FDA). The FDA was gradually taken over by the patent medicine industry – the very industry it was assigned to regulate. Patent medications that are hazardous or deadly have been approved by the FDA.

Consequences

When you remove a substance from a plant, the other parts of the plant that act as controls to reduce harmful side effects are missing.

> **Synergy of life:** "The whole is greater than the sum of the parts, and the parts require the other parts to realize their full potential."

When a synthetic drug is made, usually from coal tar or petroleum, it may mimic nature, but a synthetic substance is not recognized by the body and may not enhance but rather decrease the quality of healing.

Because not every drug can be tested with every other drug in every individual, a person taking more than one drug at a time becomes a walking experiment. If this would be harmful to a well person, imagine the effects on an unhealthy body.

Drugs may kill bacteria, bringing responses that may relieve symptoms; however, the problem that caused the symptoms is still there. And as germs adapt to their environment, they become more resistant to the drugs that used to kill them. In addition, antibiotics, for example, go after *all* bacteria, good as well as harmful. Treating symptoms is never enough to correct the cause.

Points to Ponder

- Americans are not getting the best advice for preventing and treating disease. There is not enough data to make informed choices about foods, drugs, health remedies and nutritional supplements.

- Medical colleges are funded by or owned by drug companies. So doctors prescribe according to their training.

- Doctors are not trained in nutrition nor how to balance a diet. They are trained to administer drugs. At the most, physicians receive a two hour course on nutrition. To improve your heath, you must learn how to prevent sickness and disease. That comes through education.

- Caffeine is an addictive drug that flushes magnesium out of the body. Without magnesium there is no assimilation of calcium.

- Decaf turns to formaldehyde in the transverse colon.

- Cola is better known as battery acid.

- Carbonation dissolves teeth and bones.

- One drug company's motto is "From the womb to the tomb."

"Drugs cannot get rid of disease because they cannot build or rejuvenate tissue as foods can. Drugs have their place, but only food can replace old worn-out tissue with new." *The Chemistry of Man, Bernard Jensen, PhD p 106*

Herbs, Drugs, and Doctors

Most natural therapies are safer with fewer side effects than most patent medications. Drugs and natural medicines can still potentially interact in dangerous ways. Three million adults who are 65 years or older who risk potential adverse interactions.

The reason we allow doctors to poison us with harmful drugs is because we trust in their knowledge and education more than we do in our own senses. Doctors treat symptoms, not the person, and may be dismissive and offensive when holistic health is mentioned. This is why 70% of people who use alternative medicine do not tell their doctor, but physicians are aware that the use of complementary and alternative medical practices is rapidly on the rise.

"One of the most impressive statements I have ever heard was made by one of the doctors at my graduation exercises. He said: 'One of these days, my colleagues, you will be called in on many cases. You will find that 85-90% of these cases will be acute. According to the law of 'cure,' you will find that these acute cases get well of their own accord.' Then he added, 'but for God's sake, do something about it so that you will get the credit.'" *The Science and Practice of Iridology, Dr. Bernard Jensen, DC, ND p 45*

People seek alternative medicines for prevention or treatment of chronic and progressive diseases, especially when traditional medicine offers no cures. In fact, patent medicines can have dangerous side effects that are often worse than the original complaint or condition.

You must take personal responsibility for your health. Look for natural therapies whenever possible. Tell your general practitioner about your herbal supplementation and/or natural remedies. If your physician is not willing to work with you, find a physician who will and who is knowledgeable about natural medicine for a proper diagnosis of your condition

"They will pick up snakes with their hands; and when they drink deadly poison, it will not hurt them at all; they will place their hands on sick people, and they will get well." *Mark 16:18 NIV*

Judging whether a food or substance is good for us is a God-given instinct. Studies have found, for example, that many oncologists do not or would not take chemotherapy if they themselves were diagnosed with cancer. Unfortunately, most of us have been trained to ignore these signals.

HYDROGEN PEROXIDE

The hydrogen peroxide molecule (H_2O_2) is basically water (H_2O) with an extra oxygen atom attached. Hydrogen peroxide kills bacteria, viruses, yeast, parasites. Your own white blood cells (the body's first and best defense against any infection) produce hydrogen peroxide to kill invading germs. When hydrogen peroxide is released against germs, it *oxidizes* them. Even over-the-counter H_2O_2 is a better alternative to the high cost of drugs that condemns millions to death every year.

ASPIRIN

Aspirin is a coal tar product. Put an aspirin in a teaspoon, and hold a lighter under it. You will see a black sticky substance, salicylic acid, which is some of the residue your colon holds onto and will eventually block mineral uptake. Willows plants with natural salicin are the alternative choice to aspirin.

A University of Maryland Medical Center did a study on blood platelet clumping. It reveled that 64% of daily aspirin-takers were at risk of coronary events, which can lead to heart attacks.

If this University of Maryland study is correct, a daily aspirin INCREASES the risk of coronary events in people with healthy (and normal) LDL cholesterol levels of 180, 200, or more.

REMEDIES FOR COLD OR FLU

At the first sign of cold or flu symptoms, support your body's immune system with the following nutritional supplements.

Colloidal Silver

Take two dropperfuls of colloidal silver (5-10 ppm potency) every two to four hours for an acute infection, decreasing to every six to eight hours as symptoms subside. Swish the solution in your mouth for 60 seconds before swallowing to enhance absorption.

Research indicates that colloidal silver may be a natural antibiotic and preventive against bacterial, viral, and fungal infections. It may also help against sinus and ear infections.

While studying regeneration of limbs, spinal cords, and organs in the late 1970s, Robert O. Becker, MD, author of The Body Electric, discovered that silver ions promote bone growth and kill surrounding bacteria.

Colostrum

Take 500 mg twice a day, in capsule form, on an empty stomach. Make sure it contains only colostrum or acidophilus, as other ingredients can interfere with absorption. This milk is produced by all mammals after delivery of their newborn and is crucial to initiating the immune response. A number of studies have found colostrum to be helpful in the treatment of diseases such as rheumatoid arthritis, endometriosis, allergies, colds, and herpes.

Echinacea

Echinacea works by increasing the number of phagocytes, specialized cells that surround and engulf pathogens, and stimulates other "killer" cells such as T and B lymphocytes. Echinacea sometimes can stop a cold that is just starting as well as make colds shorter and less severe. Take 10-30 drops of a 1% echinacoside liquid extract three times daily.

Take Echinacea no longer than eight weeks at a stretch, and do not use it at all if you have an autoimmune condition.

Mineral-Buffered Vitamin C

Start with moderate doses – 500 to 1,000mg – one to three times daily. Work up to as much as 5,000 to 10,000mg (5-10 grams) a day. Level off and decrease your dosage when you reach "bowel tolerance" (loose stools).

Vitamin C is antiviral and antibacterial. It increases antibody levels and enhances your immune system. It very useful for shortening the course of colds and flu.

Name These Herbal Remedies

1. This remedy is used as a liver or kidney tonic, as a diuretic, and for minor digestive problems. Its leaves can be eaten raw. It can be made into wine.

2. This herb has been used to treat rheumatoid arthritis, menopausal discomforts, and PMS. It's also been used during pregnancy to shorten labor.

3. This is used to prevent dental plaque and to treat urinary tract infections.

4. This remedy is used primarily as a laxative, is thought to potentially ease menopausal hot flashes, and may even benefit people with heart disease. (Hint: It can also be eaten in salads.)

5. Used as a spice, this remedy treats heartburn, stomach ulcers, and gallstones. It can also be made into a paste and applied directly on the skin to treat eczema.

6. Belonging to the legume family, this remedy has historically been used for respiratory problems. It is used to ease menopausal symptoms, to treat high cholesterol, osteoporosis, and symptoms of prostate enlargement.

7. Used in cooking, this remedy eases motion sickness and nausea caused by chemotherapy. It is also used to treat joint and muscle pain.

8. Another well-known cooking herb, the plant that this remedy comes from is in the lily family. It's used to treat high cholesterol, heart disease, high blood pressure, and also to prevent stomach and colon cancers.

9. Also known as "goat weed," this herbal remedy is used to treat depression, sleep disorders, and nerve pain.

10. Used in China for more than 400 years, this remedy may suppress the immune system, fight inflammation, and have anti-cancer effects.

ANSWERS:

1. Dandelion
2. Evening Primrose Oil
3. Cranberry
4. Flax seed
5. Turmeric
6. Red Clover
7. Ginger
8. Garlic
9. St. John's Wort
10. Thunder God Vine

Source: *National Center for Complementary and Alternative Medicine*

CHAPTER 9

Water

Water, Water Everywhere

Water is the most significant nutrient, because it is essential for life. You can live as long as two months without food, but you will die within a few days without water.

Water is absorbed almost immediately, and the body holds it both inside (intracellular) and outside (extracellular) the cells.

WATER FACTS

- 75% of Americans are chronically dehydrated.

- In 37% of Americans, the thirst mechanism is so weak that it is often mistaken for hunger.

- Even MILD dehydration will slow down metabolism as much as 3%.

- One glass of water will shut down midnight hunger pangs for almost 100% of the dieters studied in a University of Washington study.

- Lack of water is the #1 trigger of daytime fatigue.

- Preliminary research indicates that 8 -10 glasses of water a day could significantly ease back and joint pain for up to 80% of sufferers.

- A mere 2% drop in body water can trigger fuzzy short-term memory, trouble with basic math, and difficulty focusing on the computer screen or on a printed page.

- Merely drinking 5 glasses of water daily decreases the risk of colon cancer by 45%, slashes the risk of breast cancer by 79%, and makes you 50% less likely to develop bladder cancer.

- Large quantities of water consumed at one time over strain the muscles of the digestive tract.

A VALUABLE OXYGEN SOURCE

- Most of the oxygen in the body comes from water.

- The consumption of carbonated beverages produces more carbon dioxide than oxygen.

- Boiled water is oxygen deficient, and distilled water is dead water.

- Water promotes the ability to dissolve nutrients in the blood and body fluids.

- Water also acts as a solvent for body waste – urea, carbon dioxide and various toxins.

- The body of a newborn baby is approximately 80-85% water.

- Dehydration slowly occurs, but as we age, dehydration rates increase.

- Water accounts for only 70% of body weight by the time of middle age. This loss of water continues in all the tissues of the body, producing signs of age degeneration such as wrinkles.

Types of Water

SPRING WATER

This water comes from an underground source of generally pure water that rises to the surface as a spring. Most are protected to keep them pure, yet natural impurities such as arsenic, fluoride, radon, and uranium can enter the water.

MINERAL WATER

Mineral water must contain a minimum of 250 parts per million of dissolved minerals, mostly calcium and magnesium. A number have higher levels of fluoride as well.

ARTESIAN WATER

This is water that originates from an aquifer, a deep underground flow of water. As with mineral water it can contain some contaminants but less than surface water.

SPARKLING WATER

This water is naturally carbonated. Most contain added carbonation due to the loss of the natural "fizz" during processing. Many have high levels of fluoride.

DISTILLED WATER

This is water prepared by boiling the water and then condensing the steam. This removes all contaminants except the volatile gases, which need to be removed by carbon filtration. Minerals can be added back to the water. Adding ¼ teaspoon of good sea salt per liter will remineralize the water.

Consumption of distilled water in large quantities washes waste products and toxins from the body, destroys germs, and cleanses the organism with the aid of chlorine. Prolonged use of distilled water is not advised because it also draws mineral salts from the body. It is more indicated in cases of arthritis, gout, rheumatism, and hardening and deposits in the body. Distilled water may cause you to lose hair. Considerable quantities of distilled water increase urination helping to remove acids, toxins, and other harmful products. (The Chemistry of Man, Bernard Jensen PhD, p. 153)

REVERSE OSMOSIS WATER

Reverse osmosis water was thought to be the best for purifying drinking water. Recent studies, however, reveal that mold and fungus may be found in the filtration process. It has also been discovered that reverse osmosis steals minerals from the body.

BOTTLED WATER

Bottled water is costly and may not be safer or healthier than tap water. Studies have found that tap water tends to have lower bacterial counts than bottled. Some bottled waters are merely tap water, and are out of line with standards. More than 150 million Americans drink bottled water.

Plastic containers are not as weighty as glass but can affect the water. Clear polyethylene plastic should have a triangle with number 2 or 4. Do not freeze your plastic water bottles with water as it releases dioxin, a health hazard.

Bottled water is not always regulated by the FDA. The FDA standards apply only to bottled water that is distributed nationally – not regionally. However, an estimated 60% to 70% of the bottled water we buy in the US is regional and thus, exempt from FDA control.

The news media recently reported that trace amounts of a whole pharmacopeia of medications, antibiotics to antidepressants to oral contraceptives, were detected in the water supply of major cities – the water supply that some bottling factories get their water from – and further, that the bottles themselves leach harmful chemicals into the water. There is also the environmental impact of all those plastic bottles tossed in the trash to consider.

Theoretically bottled water is regulated at the state level, but only 40 of the 50 states actually do so, and even those have limited or no resources for actual enforcement. Check with the water commission (Bureau of Water Quality Assurance or Water Resources Control Board) for the state's requirements.

CARBONATED AND SELTZER WATER

The FDA has some vague sanitation rules about these products but with no specific limits on contaminants, and less than 50% of states require water in these categories to meet regular interstate bottled water standards.

TAP WATER

Bottled water and tap water are regulated by entirely different federal agencies. Tap water is always regulated by the EPA, but do not assume that the water that comes from your kitchen faucet is 100% safe. The EPA sets standards for about 90 contaminants in drinking water, including the protozoan pathogens giardia and cryptosporidium (both of which can produce gastrointestinal illness like diarrhea and vomiting) plus other contaminants like lead, asbestos, and arsenic – but the testing and reporting is done by the water companies, themselves, and on the honor system.

According to a report by the environmental action group, National Resources Defense Council, out of 19 cities tested, about one-fourth rated poor for water quality and compliance. A 2005 report by another consumer advocacy group, the Environmental Working Group, found that tap water in 42 states contained many contaminants that were dangerous, if not technically illegal. According to the report, of the 141 contaminants identified, 52 are linked to cancer, 41 to reproductive toxicity, 36 to developmental defects, and 16 to immune system damage.

For more facts check out www.epa.gov/safewater.com.

Private wells that supply fewer than 25 people are not under government jurisdiction, so well owners should test annually since the EPA doesn't check individual residences. Local health departments can help provide guidance about well water quality.

EPA's Safe Drinking Water Hotline: 800-426-4791

Environmental Working Group: www.ewg.org

Natural Resources Defense Council: www.nrdc.org

Cold Water Versus Hot Water

COLD WATER

- Does not reduce body temperature
- Reduces the pulse rate and increases arterial tension
- Remains in the stomach longer than hot water

- Should not be consumed with a meal because it slows digestion
- Increases the secretion of digestive juices more than hot water
- Urine flow is increased by cold water
- Consumption increases fat oxidation only in warm-blooded, stout people

HOT WATER

- Reduces body temperature by converting heat into perspiration
- Passes rapidly through the stomach
- No more than 3 oz of hot water at a meal aids digestion
- Reduces urine flow
- Increase perspiration and evaporation
- Reduces fat metabolism and leads to leanness eventually
- Diabetic patients benefit by hot water

How Much Water?

Drink up to, but not more than, 1 gallon of water per day. It may tend to wash out minerals.

Rule of thumb: ½ your body weight in number of ounces per day.

Let the Drinker Beware!

FLUORIDE

"We would not purposely add arsenic to the water supply. And we would not purposely add lead. But we do add fluoride. The fact is that fluoride is more toxic than lead and just slightly less toxic than arsenic." *Dr. John Yiamouyiannis, esteemed scientist*

"I am appalled at the prospect of using water as a vehicle for drugs. Fluoride is a corrosive poison that will produce serious effects on a long-term basis. Any attempt to use water this way is deplorable." *Dr. Charles Gordon Heyd, past president of the American Medical Association*

The ingestion of fluoride has been linked to birth defects, osteoporosis, and the propensity to increase lead absorption in children. Researchers have discovered that fluoride creates a brittle shell on the outside of bones and teeth, while creating a porous situation on the inside, and studies that link increased fracture rates and fluoride have been reported by both the "New England Journal of Medicine" and "The Journal of the American Medical Association". Furthermore, the brittle shell over teeth has led some dental professionals to believe that tooth decay is not lower in fluoridated communities.

Holland banned fluoridation in 1976 and modified its constitution so that it could never again be introduced. France rejected fluoridation in 1980 because the Chief of Public Health declared it was too dangerous.

WATER BOTTLES

Of course drinking water is an excellent habit to develop to rehydrate the kidneys, support weight loss, energize muscles, keep skin looking younger, and stimulate brain cells. Before you purchase bottled water, however, keep the following in mind.

Bottles have a number on the bottom to be used as a guide to plastic safety. Certain plastics leach chemicals that have been linked to risks – including improper brain development in fetuses, infants, and children – into food and water.

Never drink water from a bottle labeled with a #3, 6, or 7.

Plastics with #3 have been linked to cancers, such as breast and prostate cancer, as well as to hormonal imbalances.

Plastics with #6 interfere with hormones.

Plastics with #7 (of the greatest concern) have been linked to breast and ovarian cancer. The U.S. Center for Disease Control and Prevention discovered that toxins from #7 had leached into 90% of the people tested.

Plastics with #1, 2, 4, or 5 can be used for drinking water, but should be discarded after the first use. Recycle these bottles, and be conscious of the environment.

Choose a bottle with the recycling symbol #2 HDPE (high-density polyethylene), #4 LDPE (low-density polyethylene), or #5 PP (poly-propylene). These bottles do not leach.

Do not drink out of any plastic bottle after it has been exposed to heat (including from the sun) as it will leach toxins into your drink.

Glass water bottles are my personal preference. The drawbacks of using glass are breakage and leakage! Insulated bottle pouches are easy to find and help to reduce these problems.

Check the recycling numbers on all of your plastic containers, not just those used for water. I suggest you start swapping out all toxic plastics for glass containers.

CHAPTER 10

Sweeteners

Sugar Is Toxic

Refined sugar lacks proteins, vitamins, and minerals. Proteins, vitamins and minerals are present in the original form – the sugar beet or the cane plant – in quantities sufficient to metabolize the carbohydrate in the plants. However, refined sugar has been stripped of its life force and is a pure, refined carbohydrate. Dr. William Coda Martin classified refined sugar as a poison, not really a food but more of a chemical, which is difficult to utilize and digest.

Refined starches and carbohydrates provide only empty calories and are considered lethal. Concentrated carbohydrate excesses, especially refined sweets, are harmful to the endocrine glands. When consumed every day, sugar produces a continuously over-acid condition and will eventually result in dental caries, joint problems, and mental difficulties.

When you are limited in your food choices (i.e. a breakfast or luncheon business meeting, traveling, dinner parties, etc.), try to eat a protein with the meal. Protein will help to slow down the sugar imbalances and reduce the insulin/glucagon effect.

"When you enter a town and are welcomed, eat what is set before you." *Luke 10:8 NIV*

Also remember to pray over your food. You will be amazed at how it changes the molecular structure and chemistry of the food.

Natural Sweeteners

Any type of sweetener is on the higher end of the glycemic index. Occasionally you can replace man-made, processed, empty calories with the following list of natural sweeteners.

SUCANAT

Sucanat (**SU**gar **CA**ne **NAT**ural) is organically grown, freshly-squeezed sugar cane juice. It is highly nutritious because the molasses is not removed. You can replace white sugar and brown sugar (white sugar with a bit of molasses added to give texture and color) with sucanat. In hot or cold water, it is a refreshing beverage. A teaspoon of dried Sucanat will even relieve hiccups.

UNPASTEURIZED HONEY

Although not as high in vitamins and minerals as sucanat, honey is a useful natural sweetener. Natural, raw honey is a naturally pure substance. Honey contains trace minerals and enzymes and has antibacterial properties that will help with your overall health. It has the plant enzyme, amylase, which is concentrated in the pollen of flowers and is effective in predigestion of starchy foods. If you spread raw honey on a piece of bread and allow it to sit for 15 minutes, the honey will immediately begin to break down the starches in the bread.

Most commercial honey has been pasteurized, heated for up to 24 hours to prevent it from turning hard or hazy. In 1930, the German Honey Ordinance ordered that honey could not be sold for table use unless the enzyme, amylase, was intact; not so in North America.

Honey is more frugal, safer, and handier than supplements, cosmetics, ointments, antibiotics, and prescription drugs.

- Replace white sugar in all your baked goods. Reduce the liquid in the recipe by ¼ cup for each cup of honey. Cut honey's natural acidity by adding ½ teaspoon of baking soda for each cup. Reduce the baking temperature by 25°F to prevent muffins and cakes from over browning.

- Drizzle over fruit or grapefruit halves, then put it in the broiler for about two minutes.

- Spread over toast, alone or with melted butter.

- Use a teaspoon with four cups of warm water for shine treatment for your hair. Comb the mixture through your hair after a shampoo. Dry as normal.

- Soothe sore throats and clear a cough while killing dangerous bacteria in the digestive tract. "Honey and eucalyptus" cough lozenges work. Honey stops the cough and soothes the throat, while eucalyptus cools and cuts mucous. Put a quarter cup of honey into a jar, add a couple of tablespoons of lemon juice or vinegar, and take a teaspoon of this every two to three hours. Sooth and clear up laryngitis using the same concoction.

- A honey drink is better than caffeine. Add a tablespoon of honey to a cup of hot water, and drink up. Use vinegar or lemon juice for an even healthier boost.

- Honey will help rid hay fever symptoms if you chew the wax cappings from a honeycomb. Chewing this wax also has been said to be helpful in controlling sinus problems. Taking a teaspoon of local honey is more effective for some allergy sufferers.

- For a facial for acne or oily skin: Use a tablespoon of ground oatmeal (put oatmeal in your blender for a few seconds), add a tablespoon of honey and a few drops of water to help mix it. Wash your face, then spread this mixture on it, and relax for at least 10 minutes. Remove with a cloth or facial tissue, then rinse your face in warm water. This is especially good for psoriasis or other irritations.

- To help you sleep better, calm yourself or a child, put honey in a cup of warm milk (almond, hazelnut, goat milk) for a child. It can also be used in hot tea.

- Alternative medicine has been used honey for centuries to treat wounds because it is antibacterial. To keep minor wounds, scratches, and cuts from being infected, spread it over the area, and cover. It can be removed with warm water. It encourages healing, seals in moisture, and can prevent or lessen scars.

- Add to liquid lecithin or wheat germ oil for an effective and inexpensive lip balm.

- Try a teaspoonful for heartburn. It has been proven to reduce gastric acid, and it is effective against gastroenteritis, caused by salmonella, e. coli, and shigella.

- Honey will relieve the heat of a sunburn.

- For fruit stains on clothing, rub with honey before placing in the wash.

- Honey can contain spores that cause infant botulism. Never give honey (or corn syrup or other natural sweeteners) to an infant or a child under one year old as it is very dangerous to the immature system of babies.

Caution: See your doctor in the case of a serious medical problem.

FROZEN JUICE CONCENTRATE

All frozen concentrates have been pasteurized but are healthier for sweetening a sauce or salad dressing than white sugar. Pineapple, apple, and orange concentrates are excellent for sweetening salad dressings or perking up fresh juice combinations, making Popsicles®, and for baking. A tablespoon of frozen pineapple concentrate will liven up a fruit salad.

DATES AND RAISINS

"Strengthen me with raisins, refresh me with apples, for I am faint with love." *Solomon 2:5 NIV*

Take a handful of dates, raisins, or figs, and place them in your blender with ½ cup of water. Blend for 10 minutes or until desired consistency. This recipe will create a caramel pudding-like substance that is good for you! It can be used for salad dressings, topping for fruit salad, creating healthy desserts, and baking.

FRUCTOSE

Although assimilated into the body more slowly than white sugar, fructose has essentially the same nutritional value. Fructose is the sugar that is primarily found in fruit. It breaks down more slowly because it does not use insulin, but it is broken down by an enzyme in the bowel. Fructose sugar looks identical to white sugar but is significantly sweeter. It is a safer sugar to use for diabetics, hyperglycemics, and hypoglycemics. Fructose is certainly more desirable than common sugar but is still devoid of nutrients. Use sparingly.

DATE SUGAR

Date sugar is made from ground, dehydrated dates and is not really just a sugar. It is rich in nutrients and is metabolized more slowly since it contains all the vitamins, minerals, and fiber found in the whole fruit. In most recipes, especially baking, it can be used in equal parts for sugar. It is also a great substitute for brown sugar. It cannot be used to sweeten beverages because the tiny pieces do not dissolve.

BLACKSTRAP MOLASSES

When sugar is extracted from the cane, blackstrap molasses is the residual syrup that remains at the very end of the sugar extraction process. It contains the lowest sugar content of the molasses but is highest in vitamins, minerals, and other nutrients. As a healthful, nutritious sweetener, it contains 258 times as much calcium as sugar.

To make a quick substitution in your baking, replace each cup of granulated sugar with 1/3 cup of molasses. Reduce the liquid in the recipe by ¼ cup for each cup of molasses you use.

STEVIA

Studies done on stevia, mostly in Japan, indicate that this is a safe herb. Natives from many countries have used this herb as a natural sweetener. They have lower rates of cancer, grow to average heights and weights, and continue to reproduce normally.

Stevia is extracted from a South American herb that is 100 to 400 times sweeter than conventional white sugar. It is available in powders and liquid extracts in the supplement section of natural product stores. It does not upset blood sugar and can assist in regulating blood-sugar levels. Some first time stevia users report an aftertaste, but with continued use, this calorie-free herb is a great tasting sugar substitute.

You can purchase stevia as whole or powdered leaf. Many tea blends contain the whole leaf. Fresh stevia leaves contain calcium, vitamin C, beta-carotene, chromium, fiber, potassium, niacin, magnesium, iron, protein, and silicon.

There are many health benefits of drinking tea made from stevia, including:

- has 5x the antioxidants of green tea (and no caffeine)
- enhances immunity and natural healing power
- kills food poisoning bacteria but does not harm useful intestinal bacteria
- kills viruses
- detoxifies chemicals
- prevents allergies
- anti-oxidizing effect
- detoxifies histamine
- digestive aid
- regulates blood sugar in people with diabetes
- inhibits the growth and reproduction of oral bacteria
- lowers incidence of colds and flu
- reduces the craving for sweets

To grow stevia in your garden, it does best in an environment that is hot, humid, and wet. Mountain Rose Herbs sells the seeds.

Once you have your fresh or dried stevia leaves, you can use them to make hot or iced tea, and to make a stevia concentrate, which you can use as a liquid sweetener.

To make tea: add 3 teaspoons stevia leaf (2 teabags) to one quart (4 cups) water. If using room temperature water, steep 4 hours. If using hot water, steep a few minutes, until desire taste. Or use room temperature water, and place it in the sun to brew for 2 hours. Add mint, ginger, lemon, or any other herbs you like.

To make Homemade Liquid Stevia Concentrate: Place 1 cup warm water in a glass jar, and add ¼ cup stevia leaf powder. Let sit 24 to 48 hours. Repeat until the liquid reaches your desired sweetness. Strain through cheesecloth. Keep refrigerated. Put some in a small dropper bottle for ease of use.

How to use stevia in place of sugar:

- 1 cup of sugar = 1 teaspoon white powdered extract, 2 tablespoons whole leaf powder, or 1 teaspoon liquid concentrate.

- 1 tablespoon sugar = 3/8 teaspoon whole leaf powder, ¼ teaspoon white powdered extract, or approximately 8 drops of liquid concentrate.

- 1 teaspoon sugar = 1/8 teaspoon whole leaf powder, one pinch or 1/16 teaspoon white powdered extract, or approximately 3-4 drops liquid concentrate.

AGAVE

The agave traditionally used in Mexico to treat illnesses is different than the agave marketed in the United States. This dark, thick agave liquid has a very strong flavor and characteristic smell with a high concentration of mineral salts such as calcium, magnesium, sodium, and potassium, as well as amino acids.

The traditional agave syrup is replaced with a more refined syrup and does not have the same life giving properties and nutrients. Commercial manufacturers decided to create a more delicate product with a more palatable flavor, and this is the agave nectar we see on store shelves.

This juice is expressed from the core of the plant and is highly processed using caustic acids, clarifiers and filtration chemicals resulting in 70-92% pure fructose. Although possibly higher in minerals than most refined sweeteners, it is not likely healthy for regular use due to its high fructose level, much higher than honey and maple syrup.

Given what we now know about the deleterious effects of fructose compared to sucrose, honey, and maple syrup would seem to be better choices than agave for home cooking.

It is extracted from agave, is 42% sweeter than white sugar but has the same caloric value and a low glycemic index (11).

XYLITOL

Xylitol is a natural sugar alcohol, not actually a sugar. The molecular structure of xylitol is a reason why many carcinogenic bacteria cannot metabolize it. Xylitol is a proven antibacterial, anti-fungal, and immune enhancer and actually improves dental properties. It tastes like sugar, but it does not spike blood sugar. It may cause diarrhea if consumed in excess.

Artificial Sweeteners

Some artificial sweeteners are carcinogenic and worse than sugar. The warning labels, "cancer causing", on saccharin still apply.

ASPARTAME

Since the 1980s, American corporations wanted to protect their profits (trillions of dollars) by keeping the truth behind aspartame's dangers hidden from the public. However, history and research concludes that aspartame, a chemical food additive, causes toxic reactions and illness to the human body.

When NutraSweet® (Equal®) was introduced for the second time in 1981, America was in a diet craze, and profits made from the revolutionized eating protocols called for a change in modern lifestyles. More than twenty years later, people are figuring out for themselves that aspartame is at the root of their health problems. Dr. H. J. Roberts, a diabetes expert, believes there is a clear scientific link between aspartame and increased incidence of brain tumors, seizure disorders, chronic headaches, and hyperactivity in children. Over 92 different health symptoms are at the root of aspartame dangers in modern disease. The use of aspartame during pregnancy and by children is one of the greatest aspartame dangers of all.

You may return all food products with aspartame, opened or unopened, to your grocer. When you tell him/her that the products make you sick, the grocer can return them to the manufacturer for a store refund. This will send a message to the grocer and to the manufacturer.

The most effective way to reverse aspartame dangers is to remove aspartame from the diet. Get back to the basics of eating and enjoying natural foods. Drink purified water, and clean up your diet as much as possible. Become aware of artificial food substitutes that are hidden in your foods, and exercise regularly. When you avoid artificial sweeteners, refined sugars and carbohydrates, and caffeine, your body will begin to detoxify and restore itself.

Below are some reported side effects from aspartame:

- Fibromyalgia symptoms
- Menstrual problems
- Multiple sclerosis symptoms
- Dizziness
- Headaches

Splenda®

Splenda® is the brand name for sucralose, a non-nutritive sweetener added to hundreds of foods and beverages in the United States. Americans are like guinea pigs in a science experiment buying products they think are better than those with sugar. There is a lack of long-term studies.

Below is a list of reactions from using Splenda. Many symptoms could have other causes; however, they apparently disappear when Splenda is removed from the diet.

Flushing or redness of the skin

Acne or acne-like rash

Burning feeling of the skin

Anxiety

Rash

Panic attacks

Itching

Feelings of food poisoning

A panicky or shaky feeling

Headache

Swelling

Seeing spots

Blisters on the skin

Mental or emotional breakdown

Unexplained crying

Feeling Faint

Dulled senses

Shaking

Welts

Altered emotional state (i.e. feeling irate, impatient, hypersensitive)

Nausea

Stomach cramps

Bloated abdomen

Dry heaves

Diarrhea

Becoming withdrawn

Trouble concentrating or staying in focus

Loss of interest in usual activities

Feeling depressed

Feeling forgetful

Vomiting

Moodiness

Seizures

I was on a flight to Texas in November, 2007 when I noticed a woman next to me intensely reading a small packet of Splenda®. I commented about the dangers of Splenda®, and the man sitting next to her looked over at me and said, "We manufacture that!" (Well... oops!)

To my surprise, they were both cordial, and the woman proceeded to share with me that very few of those who produce it actually use it! She stated that when sucralose was taken off the market, there was such a public outcry for a replacement. Splenda® was the answer to the demand.

They both commented about another item in the works that was sure to be pricey and "probably be sold only in health food stores". The product – pure cane sugar – imagine that! They even showed the packaging to me, and I just smiled. (I wonder if they realize it could possibly be good for them!)

Learn to read food labels. Examples of added sugars include:

Corn Syrup	Glucose
Dextrose	Honey
Sugar	Lactose
Syrup	Maltose
Fructose	Molasses
Fruit juice concentrates	Sucrose

Soda

One can of soda has about 10 teaspoons of sugar, is loaded with artificial food colors, sulphites, and artificial sweeteners. Appetite for healthy foods will be suppressed. Osteoporosis, obesity, tooth decay, and heart disease are linked to soda.

Makes you gain weight. One to two cans of soda a day increases the risk of being overweight or obese by 32.8%.

Increases your disease risk. Whether regular or diet, 44% are more likely to develop metabolic syndrome—a condition that greatly increases your risk for heart disease and diabetes according to a 2007 study published in the American Heart Association's journal "Circulation".

Has no nutritional value. A 20-ounce bottle of cola soda contains nearly 250 calories, no vitamins, no minerals.

Does not satisfy your thirst. Soda may make you thirstier because caffeine is a diuretic, and sugar interferes with the body's absorption of fluids. To quench your thirst, try water, herbal tea, or fruit juice.

Is bad for digestion. Soda drinkers may develop digestive distress, acid reflux, stomach inflammation, and intestinal erosion because of the phosphoric acid, which may disturb the acid-alkaline balance of the stomach.

Can be addictive. Soft-drink manufacturers add caffeine to get consumers hooked, according to a 2000 study published in the Archives of Family Medicine. Caffeine is a stimulant, and eliminating soda may create withdrawal symptoms, including fatigue, depression, irritability, tremors, sleep deprivation, and headaches.

Is not eco-friendly. An estimated 50 billion aluminum cans and plastic bottles from soft drinks get thrown into landfills every year.

Is bad for your bones and teeth. Phosphoric acid in cola prevents calcium from being absorbed. A 2006 study, published in General Dentistry, reported citric and/or phosphoric acid in soft drinks is damaging to teeth.

May cause cancer. A 2006 study from Sweden's Karolinska Institute: subjects who drank high quantities of fizzy or syrup-based soft drinks twice a day or more ran a 90% higher risk of developing pancreatic cancer.

Costs money. An average 12-ounce can costs about $1 from the vending machine, so two a day for a year adds up to $730 every year.

TEN GREAT USES FOR Coca-Cola®

1. In many states, the highway patrol carries two gallons of Coca-Cola® in the truck to remove blood from the highway after a car accident.

2. You can put a T-bone steak in a bowl of Coca-Cola® and it will be gone in two days.

3. To clean a toilet, pour a can of Coca-Cola® into the toilet bowl and let the "real thing" sit for one hour, then flush clean. The citric acid in Coca-Cola® removes stains from vitreous china.

4. To remove rust spots from chrome car bumpers: Rub the bumper with a rumpled up piece of aluminum foil dipped in Coca-Cola®.

5. To clean corrosion from car battery terminals: Pour a can of Coca-Cola® over the terminals to bubble away the corrosion.

6. To loosen a rusted bolt: Apply a cloth soaked in Coca-Cola® to the rusted bold for several minutes.

7. To remove grease from clothes: Empty a can of Coca-Cola® into a load of greasy clothes, add detergent, and run through a regular cycle.

8. Coca-Cola® will clean road haze from your windshield.

9. The active ingredient in Coca-Cola® is phosphoric acid. It has an acidic pH of 2.8, which will dissolve a nail in about 4 days.

10. The distributors of Coca-Cola® have been using it to clean the engines of their trucks for about 20 years!

To carry Coca-Cola® syrup (the concentrate), a commercial truck must use the hazardous material warning cards reserved for highly corrosive materials.

Phosphoric acid in Coca-Cola® leaches calcium from bones and is a major contributor to the rising increase in osteoporosis.

Regarding Drinks That Dissolve Your Teeth

In a study done at the University of Texas Health Science Center at San Antonio in association with the University of California at San Francisco and Indiana University in Indianapolis, Bennett T. Amaechi, PhD, associate professor of community dentistry examined the teeth of 900 children between the ages of 10 and 14 in three different areas of the country.

The study revealed that 30% of the kids had dental erosion in which the enamel on the teeth begins to erode, leaving teeth thinner, and less protected. Ironically, initially this erosion makes teeth smoother and shinier, so it is highly unlikely that people will notice the early stage of this destruction.

The erosion results from repeated exposure to certain drinks including soft drinks, fruit and sports drinks, some herbal teas, beer salts (lime-flavored salts added to beer), and fruit-flavored candies, called Lucas candies, imported from Mexico. Even healthy foods such as citrus fruits and drinks like seltzer will erode enamel. All of these are acidic – and excessive acid literally dissolves the enamel off teeth.

TO REPAIR THE DAMAGE

Cutting back on the offending beverages stops the erosion, and over time, saliva actually begins to remineralize the tooth surface, though never completely. The erosion progresses and eventually causes great sensitivity and pain if you do not stop. Teeth may begin to lose their shape. With regular dental exams, the dentist can identify the problem in time for patients to put an end to their bad habits.

Limit how often you have citrus-based drinks. Consider sipping the drinks through a straw to lessen contact with teeth. The worst possible habit is drinking sodas all day long. Also avoid brushing immediately after eating or drinking the acidic product.

Source:
Bennett T. Amaechi, PhD, associate professor of community dentistry at University of Texas Health Science Center, San Antonio

Gymnema

Gymnema works to remove the taste of the sugar. When you put it in your mouth, your taste buds do not detect any sweet flavors. Within minutes, eating a cookie tastes like eating a wad of salt and flour and is not very appetizing. It works best when taken about 10 to 15 minutes before meals.

It also works to control blood sugar levels. It has been used for over 2,000 years to treat diabetes. It will not drop your blood sugar levels enough to cause hypoglycemia, but it could happen if used with insulin or anti-diabetic drugs. In these cases, Gymnema should only be taken under professional supervision.

Gymnema is suitable for use in children, and is valuable in delaying the onset of type 1 diabetes when there is evidence of its development. Children should be given a fraction of the adult dose: Divide the child's weight in pounds by the number 130. That's the fraction of the adult dose you should use. For example, if the child weighs 65 lbs. then he would receive half the adult dose.

CHAPTER 11

Emotional Health

"Pleasant words are a honeycomb, sweet to the soul and healing to the bones." *Proverbs 16:24 NASB*

Green Wrapper and Ginger Chews

In place of candy, I kept a tub of ginger chews in my office. These chews had a double wrapper – a green cover on the outside with a white baker's paper on the inside, which would often stick to the "candy". They were tasty but spicy and enjoyed by most folks.

There was one woman, however, who made me rethink offering these ginger chews. Separating the ginger chew from the inner wrapper was, at times, a challenge, and this woman tossed the candy in the trash after her first unsuccessful attempt. She apparently felt that it was too much effort to gently pull the paper off of the candy.

On her second try, she managed to remove the inner wrapper, and she put the ginger chew into her mouth. As she bit into it, she turned up her nose, and then threw this piece in the trash, too. She decided that she did not like it, even after all the work it took to remove the wrapper.

I pondered over that woman's reaction and realized that God was saying to me that some people are like that ginger chew. The outside is a cover that is easy to remove. The inner wrapper is like some people that may be "wrapped too tight", not allowing anyone to get close enough to know them. And then some people are like the spicy ginger chew – after we struggle to unwrap their "cover", their "bite" is hard to take, so we spit them out.

A few days later, I stepped outside to feel the warmth of the April sun after a gentle spring morning rain. On the ground was a discarded green wrapper from one of the ginger chews. The green wrapper had now turned blue.

I am reminded that in life some people are mistreated, abused, discarded, or may experience a downpour of events in their lives. They become bitter and closed to avoid painful reminders. But the green wrapper had turned a special, pretty blue hue. It is our choice how we view life and to look for new possibilities and new colors in our own lives.

I believe that circumstances teach us and make us better people. That which does not break us, makes us. Allow God to make something beautiful out of your life in spite of your circumstances. Ask him to reveal His purpose for your life.

"...all things work together for good for those who... are called according to His purpose." *Romans 8:28 NET Bible*

Stress

Small doses of stress can keep you on your toes. Chronic stress everyday may have a serious impact on your health and well-being.

Stress is your body's response to:

- a parking ticket, a missed bus, or a hectic day at work
- a family argument, a tight budget, or a snooty sales clerk
- a divorce, the loss of a loved one, trying to fit time in for family and work

- feeling helpless and hopeless after hearing about family or friends who are ill or in a crisis

- anticipating Christmas schedules with financial obligations, rehearsals, and performances

Stress producers:

- negative thoughts – the most potent toxin

- food is in second place

Stress management tools:

- exercise

- deep breathing

- prayer and meditation

- decrease stress and anxiety

- improve your overall health

ATTITUDES OF THE MIND

"The attitude of the mind works for or against your well-being. It is an accepted fact that close to 80-90% of all illness begins in the brain – may I dare say 100%? You see, the brain is an electrical generator in its own right. The total body receives this electricity. Yet there is one organ that is probably more dependant upon the brain's electricity than any other. That organ is the liver. The liver uses the electricity for generating the initial magnetic attraction for the uptake of mineral energy. Without the electric flow from the brain, the magnetic properties of the liver are interfered with.

Anything that short circuits the brain's delivery of electricity to the liver will set the stage for degenerative changes in the liver, which will, in turn, affect the rest of the body. The greatest causes of interference to the brain's electrical flow to the liver are hate, bitterness, worry, fear, lust, and self-centeredness. These are the mental exercises that interfere with the flow of electricity from the brain to the organs, especially the liver, and set the stage for the initiation of close to 90% of degenerative disease. In order, then, to accomplish the proper on-going improvements in wellness, I have discovered that it is valuable to incorporate some mental-spiritual introspection. I have realized that the past and present, if not dealt with according to true principle, will short circuit and undermine my purpose and affect my desire of perfect health and well-being." *Biologic Ionization As Applied to Human Nutrition Dr. A.F. Beddoe pg. 239*

In order to accomplish improvements in wellness, it is valuable to incorporate some mental and spiritual introspection. If you do not deal with the past, the present will short circuit and undermine your life purpose and affect your health and well-being.

Dr. Masaru Emoto, author of "The True Power of Water", demonstrated how water can be changed by affixing a written statement, verbal expression, or suggestive intention upon a container of distilled water. Using Kirlian photography he was able to capture a visual frame of the effects on the water molecules. The study is quite fascinating, and I would suggest viewing the YouTube video, "Dr. Masaru Emoto's Water Molecule Experiments". The comment in the video imprints this message to us, "If thoughts can do that to water, imagine what our thoughts can do to us." Our bodies are about 90% water and our thoughts are powerful to heal or to harm!

ATTITUDES TOWARD FOOD

Eating may act as stress therapy for you. When your appetite is sparked by emotional stimuli, you have stressful thoughts generating physiological reactions. This pattern can lead you to habitual eating, and when you feel guilt about this outcome, the food you eat to feed an emotional need can have greater physiological effects on your body than food you eat just to sustain life.

Solutions and Suggestions:

- Don't eat when you are angry, sad, scared, or anxious. These emotions all shut down digestion. It is better not to eat at all when in this state.

- When we eat sugar, our immune system can be depressed for up to six hours. This is the exact same effect as when we are angry.

- Step away from hunger – get away from your kitchen and other places that you normally associate with food. Take a walk or call a friend on the telephone.

- Regular periods of rest are important and crucial to the health of your body and soul.

- Sleep is an absolute, undeniable necessity of life.

- Take a vacation each year. If you cannot get away for a lengthy vacation, taking an extended weekend will sometimes act to help restore those frazzled nerves.

- Every working creature needs a Sabbath rest. That includes people, animals, and even the soil! Besides giving us the night for regular sleep, the Creator programmed people and animals to rest completely every seventh day. When we try to change His design, things start to unravel. Even the Creator rested on the seventh day.

Consider a study that compared two identical farming soils. One was farmed continuously for eight years while the other was allowed to stand fallow, meaning that it wasn't farmed. The soil from the field that wasn't allowed to rest contained 1,097 parts per million (ppm) nutritional solids, while the fallow, or "rested", field soil yielded 2,871 ppm of nutritional solids!

In times of anger or frustration, the following prayer can help:

> "Father God, I thank You for sustaining me today. I thank You that You are made perfect in my weakness. Your grace is sufficient for me. I thank You that Your steadfast love never ceases and Your mercies are new every morning. You say in Your Word that mourning may come for a night, but the new day will bring gladness. Bless me with a healing night's sleep. Restore unto me the joy of my salvation. Help me to stay on the path that leads to life."

THE FIVE EMOTIONS OF STRESS

1. Sorrow

Life events such as: losings things we had, never receiving things we anticipated, traumas, serious illness, loss of loved ones, setbacks and disappointments, or life not turning out as we anticipated. Sorrow can make us feel incomplete. In its most severe state, we lose the will to go on.

2. Fear

As a direct result of sorrow, we experience fear. Fear of experiencing another loss; fear of being rejected by others because of our perceived deficiencies or inadequacies; fear of being unable to live up to what is expected of us.

3. Anger

Because of sorrow and fear, we may begin to feel anger, even in the form of guilt or shame. When anger is turned inward, it becomes depression. If left unresolved, this anger can ruin relationships, careers, marriages, business opportunities and your health.

4. Unworthiness

All of the previous emotions lower your self-esteem and produces feelings of unworthiness. Your motivation to try new things can decrease because you have less and less confidence in your abilities.

5. Worry

Finally, you begin to worry and over-think, creating feelings of anxiety. As your mind fills with worry, your ability to perform tasks, interact with others, and sleep decreases.

If these emotions are unchecked, the downward spiral continues, and each sorrow creates deeper struggles with these emotions. When life hands you unexpected and troubling events or the rigors of work, family, and relationships seem overwhelming, it is time to reassess.

The Benefits of Color on Mind and Body

Chromotherapy, or color therapy, is a form of energy medicine based on the belief that the human body is comprised of energy fields. In other words, color is energy that can be very therapeutic.

Colors are used to inspire, used for creativity, and used to balance moods, feelings, and emotions. For someone who lacks a specific color, more color may be needed. For someone who has too much of one color, the opposite color is utilized.

Using and avoiding certain colors is a way of self-expression; it sheds light on our personality. The following colors and their descriptions may resonate with your personality or help explain why you make the choices you do.

ORANGE

Orange is warm and cheering, it facilitates a feeling of security and is helpful to the nervous system and the mind. It stimulates creative thinking and enthusiasm. Sociable, dynamic and independent people prefer orange.

Use orange for encouragement, optimism, and energy. Think orange when needing to be kind or to receive kindness.

Orange is associated with success, abundance, prosperity, achieving business-goals, investments, and success in legal matters.

The kidneys and bladder are supported by the color orange.

YELLOW

Yellow encourages intellectual comprehension, and stimulates the pancreas, liver, and gallbladder. It is the color of the sun and represents cheerfulness and a sunny disposition. Yellow can cheer up the depressed and melancholy.

Yellow strengthens the nerves and the mind and is used for mental clarity, concentration, memorizing, and tests. When speaking and writing, or when traveling, use yellow.

An aversion to yellow may mean that you are emotionally disappointed and bitter (lemons are yellow).

RED

People with a need for personal freedom prefer red. They are temperamental and ambitious. Red also represents warmth, energy, and stimulation.

Red is associated with passionate love and sex (Valentine's Day), assertiveness and aggressiveness (anger), revolt and revolution (i.e. international symbols and flags that project courage, strength, and power), heart and blood circulation (Red Cross).

Someone who has an aversion to red may be over-active, too impulsive, or hot-tempered.

GREEN

Green suggests psychological and emotional harmony and balance and a longing for a safe home and family-life – a dislike of conflicts. It brings peace, rest, hope, comfort and nurturing, calmness, and harmony. People who prefer green have an interest in nature, plants, fellowmen, children and animals, health and healing, and a natural and plain life.

A person with an aversion to green may be more interested in independence and self-development than in a warm family life, and they may prefer to keep a certain distance in (sexual) relationships.

BLUE

People who prefer blue keep a certain distance, but give calm and practical help. They are faithful and loyal, and have a sense for order, logic, and rational thinking. Blue is for peace and tranquility, calmness, truth, wisdom, justice, counsel, guidance, understanding, patience, loyalty and honor, sincerity, devotion, healing, femininity, prophetic dreams, and protection during sleep and can be used for speech or communication such as wearing a blue scarf around the neck.

A person who has an aversion to blue may be very disciplined, a strong career-oriented worker, and may have a clear direction for their life goals.

VIOLET/PURPLE

Violet or purple soothes mental and emotional stress and counteracts depression and negativity. It is used for inspiration, meditation, and compassion. Leonardo da Vinci proclaimed that you can increase the power of meditation ten-fold by meditating under the gentle rays of violet, as found in church windows.

A person who has an aversion to violet or purple may have very serious attitudes towards life and may have a tendency to reject everything with regards to anything unnatural or unrealistic.

BLACK

Black is a color for extremes – everything, nothing. It symbolizes seriousness, darkness, depression, death, mourning, mystery, secrecy, occultism, and nothingness as the source of all creation.

People who trust themselves prefer black.

WHITE

White is the perfect color. It is in all colors, in perfect balance and harmony and symbolizes innocence, purity, virginity, cleanliness, freshness, simplicity, and truth. White is cleansing.

A person who has an aversion to the color white is solely interested in 'realistic' and tangible things, not in illusions or things that are beyond seeing or understanding.

The Power of Breath

Deep breathing calms the mind, creates a sense of well being, and leads to health. When you are angry or upset, a familiar expression comes to mind, "Take a deep breath." Notice how you are breathing then, if you are breathing at all! Our emotions are directly linked to our breathing.

Breathing is a vital and basic function, yet many of us pay little attention to our breath. We have never learned how to breathe correctly. Learning to breathe properly can greatly improve your health and reduce the impact of stress on the body.

When we breathe deeply, the impact of negative emotions on our bodies is greatly reduced. Every organ in our bodies needs oxygen to function properly. Learning to breath properly will oxygenate our blood so that our organs begin to function better.

BREATHING TECHNIQUES

Try this exercise: Close your eyes, and notice how you are breathing. Notice if your breathing is deep or shallow. Also notice what part of your torso you are breathing into. Does your belly move when you breathe? Does your rib cage expand?

To get a complete breath, breathe into three areas of the torso:

Step One – Belly Breath

To begin, sit up straight and tall (sitting in a straight back chair with your feet firmly on the ground works well), and place your hand on your belly. Exhale fully while pulling your belly in to expel all of the stale air out of your lungs. Once all of the air is out, relax your belly. Notice how the belly automatically wants to expand as the air comes in. Let the belly blow up like a balloon as the air comes in. Continue breathing into the belly for a few more rounds. The belly goes in as the breath comes out, and the belly goes out as the breath comes in.

Step Two – Thoracic Breath

Now let go of the belly breath, and place your hand on your rib cage, under your arm. As you exhale, allow the rib cage to contract. As you inhale, expand the rib cage. Let the breath be slow and full without any sense of straining. All the breathing should be through your nose. Try it a few more times.

Step Three – Upper Chest Breath

Let go of the thoracic breathing, and place your hand on the soft area above your clavicle. As you breathe in, notice how the clavicle rises slightly. Allow it to rise without lifting your shoulders. As you breathe out the clavicle falls.

It should feel like the air is coming down to an area just above the breasts. Try it for a few more rounds. Remember to breathe slowly. If you feel light headed or dizzy, increase your exhalation, and decrease your inhalation.

Step Four – Combine Three Areas into One Long Breath

Place one hand on your belly and the other on your rib cage, under your arm. Sit up nice and straight, and relax your face and jaw. Take a couple of relaxed breaths. Now exhale fully, pulling the belly in as you exhale. When you cannot exhale any further, relax the belly, and allow the air to fill your belly. The belly will blow up like a balloon. Once the belly is full, allow the air to begin to expand the rib cage. When this area is full, continue breathing in, and let the upper chest fill. The clavicle will rise slightly. As you exhale, it is just the opposite. The air goes out of your upper chest, then middle, then lower. *(It may be helpful to image a glass of water. When the water is poured into the glass, it fills the bottom, then middle, and then top. When you pour it out, it goes out of the top, then middle, then bottom. The breath is the same.)*

Learning to breathe properly is like learning to play an instrument. With time and practice, you will perfect it. Start slowly. Pay attention to the details until you can feel each area filling during a single breath. If the diaphragm and other muscles have not been used in a long time, they may need to build up strength and flexibility gradually. Practice first thing in the morning before you get out of bed. Take the pillow out from under your head, and time yourself for five minutes a day. This will dramatically impact your health and sense of well being.

BREATHING FOR HEALING

Deep breathing pumps the lymphatics, which draw fluid and toxins away from every cell in your body. This reduces inflammation and the pain that accompanies it.

Pain is usually a sign that there is a lack of oxygen to the tissues. In deep breathing exercises, pains may go away during the exercise.

Breathing is an integral part of emotional healing work. As long as a person keeps breathing, they will stay in touch with their feelings. Holding your breath stifles emotion and dulls your sense of joy and happiness, as well as causing pain.

If you're over-acidic, breathing is the fastest way to alkalize the body. In fact, breathing is the first and most important pH buffering system in the body.

Breathing helps you stay centered and relaxed and reduces your stress level. Anytime you find yourself feeling anxious, you are probably breathing shallowly. Depressed people breathe infrequently. Deep breathing calms anxiety and lifts depression, helping you cope better with a stressful situation.

The Chinese say that excessive grief damages the lungs. Dealing with suppressed grief clears the lungs. Post-nasal drip is a form of internalized crying or sadness. Older people often die of pneumonia after losing a spouse or experiencing another event that triggers deep grief. Grieving involves allowing oneself to exhale fully (e.g. to "let go").

The hiatus hernia is a sign of suppressed anger and frustration. The person can't "stomach" these intense emotions and holds them back by sucking in their breath. This is what draws the stomach up into the diaphragm. Find a safe place to connect with angry, frustrated feelings. Allow yourself to express that anger safely to help relax the stomach and bring down a hiatus hernia.

Laughter – The Best Medicine

"A cheerful look brings joy to the heart; good news makes for good health." *Proverbs 15:30 NLT*

"The human race has one really effective weapon, and that is laughter." *Mark Twain*

The release of endorphins is one of the primary benefits of exercise. Discovered in 1975, endorphins are the body's natural version of opiates such as morphine and codeine – without the addictive side effects. At least 20 different types of endorphins, secreted by the pituitary gland, have been identified, and their production is triggered by a variety of stimuli.

High endorphin levels are not only powerful pain relievers, but they also alleviate the negative effects of stress. In addition to exercise and physical activity, some foods stimulate endorphin production such as capsicum (hot peppers) and chocolate.

Dr. Don Colbert, in his book "What You Don't Know May Be Killing You", noted that research conducted by the Department of Behavioral Medicine at the UCLA Medical School into the physical benefits of happiness proved conclusively that "laughter, happiness, and joy are perfect antidotes for stress." Colbert added, "A noted doctor once said that the diaphragm, thorax, abdomen, heart, lungs — and even the liver — are given a massage during a hearty laugh."

Laughter creates good vibrations and positive feelings. People who are able to laugh at themselves put others at ease. So laugh often – it's good for your health!

"A merry heart does good, like a medicine, but a broken spirit dries the bones." *Proverbs 17:22 AKJV*

CHAPTER 12

Exercise

Exercise is for Everyone!

Exercise is important for everyone. For centuries, humans have engaged necessary exercise on the farm, at sea, or while hunting wild game. Exercising on the go is still the best way to rebuild the immune system and clear the lymphatic system.

Gather as much knowledge as possible concerning exercise and nutrition and how your body reacts. Know what your short- and long-term goals are, then apply your knowledge.

While walking or other slower-paced exercises with breaks are the best, choose the exercise best suited for your health. High-intensity aerobic exercise that seriously elevates your heart rate for long periods of time is unnatural, and such exercise can lower your immune response and create oxidation. Marathon runners face chronic ligament and joint problems, long-term degeneration of organs and tissues, and often struggle with decreased resistance to viral and bacterial infections during their peak training seasons.

A word of wisdom to parents: Children who are inactive have a five to six times greater risk of heart disease, according to researchers at the University of North Carolina at Chapel Hill.

GETTING STARTED

There is no best and only way to workout. It is all good if it works for you, but do not stay with any one method for too long. The body will adapt to any exercise routine in approximately four to six weeks, so modify your routine every three to four weeks.

Eating less food on a daily basis (calorie restriction) is not advisable, because energy sources from blood sugar, liver and muscle glycogen (sugar), and blood lipids (fat) are used to make up the caloric difference. After a few days, the liver will convert body fat to new glucose (sugar) to make up the caloric deficit.

Always perform weight training with perfect technique and form to see progress and prevent injury. Place more emphasis on why you perform the lift, not on how much weight to lift.

Manage your energy and your mind to avoid fatigue. If you have a lot of energy during a certain workout, do a few more sets, or add five minutes to your cardio routine. If you are tired, back off, or reduce the length of your cardio session.

Stay with the basics. Weight train for about 35 minutes to an hour three to four days per week, and perform cardio exercises three to four days per week for 30 to 40 minutes. Eat a little less. Take in enough protein. Drink a lot of water. Get plenty of rest. And be consistent. You will make progress. If you do not have time for all this, scale back the program, but remain consistent.

Find out how much muscle versus fat there is on your body. Do not go by height and weight recommendation charts.

Stay away from infomercial products or programs that claim to reduce body fat or to flatten your abs. These are companies looking to make a quick buck. They do not provide all the information that you require to make a wise decision. They prey on your emotion and impulse buying.

EASY DAILY WORKOUT EXERCISES

If you are not able to physically exercise for an hour three times per week, try these 10 minute exercises. Go for a short, 10 minute walk in the morning, at lunch, and at night. It all counts and will add up to a 30 minute walk. You will feel great, and it is easier than you think.

Exercising at Home

Cell Phone Marathon: There are many apps available for cell phones that will track your number of steps, especially if you are on the phone extensively. Those steps add up before you realize it when your focus is diverted. There is also wrist gadgets that motivate you to track more than just your steps. Walk around at a brisk pace while you chat. Depending on how much you talk on the phone, you could burn hundreds of calories a day this way.

Grocery Lift: Firm your arms while you carry the bags by doing bicep curls with them. Lift the bags from your sides by bending the elbows so your hands come to your shoulders. Keep your elbows in contact with your sides. Slowly lower them until they are hanging by your sides. Repeat until you get to the kitchen, and then get the next load and repeat.

Lunges: While vacuuming, firm your buttocks and legs. Do two sets of 10 repetitions on each side twice a week. As you push the vacuum handle forward, lunge forward so your knee is over your ankle. Push off your front leg as you pull the vacuum back to bring both feet together. Your right knee should be at a 90-degree angle. Hold for three seconds, and then return to the starting position by pushing up off the right leg. Repeat with the left leg.

<u>TV Tummy:</u> During commercials get down on the floor, and do a set of abdominal crunches, push ups, walk a little faster on a treadmill, or pedal on a bike. Rest through the next commercial. A lightweight dumbbell and ankle weights could also be used for arm exercises while watching TV.

Exercising At Work

<u>Leg Extensions:</u> While sitting at your desk, press your back firmly into the back of your chair. Slowly raise one leg horizontal to the floor. Hold it there for three seconds, and then slowly return it to the floor. Repeat with the other leg. Work up to 15 repetitions on each leg. Once you can do three sets of 15 repetitions easily, move to the advanced version, lifting both legs at the same time.

<u>Calf Raises:</u> Sitting in your desk chair, place both of your feet flat on the floor. Use your hands to push down on your knees. Slowly lift your heels so you are on your toes. Return to the beginning position.

<u>Side Stretch:</u> Place one hand beside your hip on the chair. Slowly extend the other arm above your head, and reach for the ceiling. Hold the stretch for 15 seconds, and repeat on the other side.

<u>Low Back and Chest Stretch:</u> Place both hands behind you, and grasp the side of your chair at shoulder height, palms facing toward the chair. Slowly lean forward, pressing the shoulders back. Slowly arch your back as you lift your chin. Return to your original position.

Muscle Toners

Improve your posture and prevent back pain with strong glut muscles. Try the following exercises.

Running/Walking: Two of the best ways to tone muscles and burn calories. Start with 20 to 30 minutes three times a week increasing the time as you build stamina.

Squats: Twice a week, do two to three sets of 10 to 15 repetitions per set to work your gluts, thighs, and back. Stand up straight with your feet hip width apart. Hold a five to 15 pounds dumbbell in each hand, palms facing up. Keep a slight arch in your lower back and your chest up, then slowly bend your knees, and push your butt back. Lower your body so that your thighs are almost parallel to the floor. Then return to the starting position by pushing through your heels to straighten your legs. *(Tip: Always keep your heels on the floor, and don't let your knees bend past your toes, or allow your upper body to bend forward.)*

StairMaster: Burn calories and target your gluts and thighs with stair climbing. Contract your gluts as you increase the level to six or above. The results appear in three weeks or sooner with just 25 to 35 minutes three to five times a week.

Butt Lifts: To lift and tighten your buttocks, do this exercise twice a week. On a padded surface or mat, do two sets of 20 repetitions on each side. Lower yourself onto all fours, elbows and knees bent and resting on the floor. Shift your body weight to your forearms for support. Bend your left knee into your chest, and then extend your leg straight behind you and parallel to the floor while squeezing your butt muscles. Keep your right knee bent and on the mat the whole time. Slowly return your leg to the starting position, and repeat with the alternate leg.

Biking: Bike 30 to 40 minutes from three to five times a week. Biking targets muscles in your butt, thighs, and hips. It is a great cardiovascular workout, too. Keep your gluts tight, and alternate between higher and lower intensity pedaling.

MAINTAINING BALANCE

Repetition should be done in a slow and fluid motion, at a rate of about four to five seconds per repetition. Begin by holding onto something, or use your arms in the exercises for security and added balance. Eventually try to perform balance exercises without support. Fix your eyes on a point straight ahead such as a painting or light switch on a wall. Maintain good posture, keep your core tight, and bend knees slightly while doing the exercises. When you can successfully perform them in a slow and controlled fashion, start to speed up the movement. This will help develop a quick reaction when you need to move fast to maintain balance, for instance when you start to slip on a wet floor.

How To Begin

With both feet on the floor, hip-width apart, do five squats, trying to get a little lower each time. Once you master the squats (after about one week), progress to balancing on a single leg. To progressively master the single-leg balance, gradually go from being assisted (holding onto something) to unassisted (letting go and balancing on your own). After mastering the single-leg balance, progress to single-leg pumps (i.e. mini squats on a single leg with upper body upright). Start with five repetitions of each exercise, and work up to 20 repetitions. This type of balance training can eventually be performed every day. Cut back on the frequency if you feel pain or see swelling.

Suggestions:

> Stand upright on one leg for 15 to 30 seconds. Then do the same on the other leg.

> Stand upright on the ball of one foot for 15 to 30 seconds, and then the other.

> Stand upright on your right leg while slowly writing your initials on the ground with your left foot in front, to the left, and behind you. Do not put any weight on the left foot while you are moving it over the surface of the ground. Now switch legs, and do the same with your right foot.

This next exercise can be performed on any 12- to 14-inch grid such as floor tiles, or you can draw the grid on a sidewalk or driveway with chalk. Stand with your right foot on the line where four tiles intersect under your arch. Touch the center of each of the four tiles that meet under your right foot with the first toe of your left foot. Take four to five seconds to move from target to target to ensure you are moving slowly and maintaining control of your body. Feel free to bend your right knee, and rotate your hips as necessary to accomplish the task. Do this both clockwise and counter-clockwise with each foot until you reach the point where you do not need to plant your moving foot for balance. Then proceed to the next level.

In this level, set yourself up the same way, and then try to touch the outside corners of the same tiles that you just touched at the center. Once you succeed, try touching the center of each of the tiles surrounding the previous four tiles. For those of you who need to be challenged further, try the outside corners of those tiles.

REBOUNDING – A LYMPHATIC MASSAGE

The rebound mini-trampoline is about 3' in diameter and 9" high. It is safe, easy to use, and can be very effective. Research has led some scientists to conclude that, "Rebound exercise is the most efficient and effective exercise yet devised by man."

Unlike jogging on hard surfaces, which puts extreme stress on certain joints, ankles, and knees, rebounding affects every joint and cell in the body equally. Vigorous exercise such as rebounding is reported to increase lymph flow by 15 to 30 times.

The lymph system bathes every cell, carries nutrients to the cell and waste products away. Without adequate movement, the cells sit in their own waste products and starve for nutrients. This contributes to arthritis, cancer, aging, and other degenerative diseases.

Doctors recommend that everyone get moderate exercise three to four times each week and walking 30 minutes daily or 60 minutes every other day. Bones become stronger with exercise. Women who exercise regularly reduce their risk of breast cancer by 72% - New England Journal of Medicine, May 1, 1997.

The lymph fluid moves through vessels that are filled with one way valves, so it always moves in the same direction. The main lymph vessels run up the legs, up the arms, and up the torso. This is why the vertical up and down movement of rebounding is so effective to pump the lymph.

With your feet in contact with the mat, bounce up and down gently. This is sufficient to give all the benefits of rebounding while strengthening the entire body. You can rebound while talking on the phone, listening to music, or watching TV. Wear running shoes to prevent slipping.

Adults should start with 5 minutes of rebounding and increase their time as fitness improves. Seniors should start with 2 minutes ten times per day, with at least 30 minutes between sessions. Hyperactive children will calm down after a few days of rebounding.

Children instinctively love the sensation of bouncing. Instead of restricting them from bouncing on a bed, buy them a mini-rebounder and help them get and stay healthy. It feels good while the body is getting help to flush toxins.

WORKOUT SCHEDULE

Try about five to 10 minutes per day, three to five days per week. In order to avoid injury, begin balance training slowly and carefully. Do not go too fast, too soon.

Don't Give Up

Tips from the President's Council on Physical Fitness to help eliminate boredom:

- Make your workouts and other exercise less structured. Change your workout to add variety.

- Find a friend or someone, even a small group who you enjoy being around. You are more likely to go with encouragement from others.

- Invest in yourself. You will feel like doing more things with more energy with family and friends. You will also feel better about yourself because your clothes fit better.

- Set a goal. Whether to lose weight or inches, have your clothes fit better or tone up the flab, or just to get healthier and feel better about yourself, make sure you set a goal, and stay focused.

ADDITIONAL TIPS

- Park farther away from the shopping center

- Take the stairs rather than the escalator or elevator

- Walk to the corner store, walk the beach, and walk through your neighborhood or the mall when the weather changes

- Burn up calories with a brisk two-mile walk. Move the arms, and stretch the legs!

- Ride a bicycle

CHAPTER 13

Environmental Hazards

Electromagnetic Fields

Electronics and electrical devices and wiring emit electromagnetic fields (EMFs) over a distance. As that distance decreases, the intensity of the radiation increases. Over the last ten years, many scientific reports have been published addressing the health risks from electromagnetic fields.

EMFs emitted from high tension wires, industrial radar, microwave beams, electric current, computers, cell phones, televisions, fluorescent lights, and other electrical appliances have been found to be dangerous to mental and physical health. Disruptive energy fields adversely impact brain wave activity, numbing or dulling our senses and perceptions.

We are an electrically charged battery carrying a life force, energy, spirit that can be measured. Sleeping or working for extensive periods within electromagnetic field zones is a constant source of stress (altering the body's polarity). Exposure can cause drowsiness, fatigue, chronic aches and pains, sleep disorders, irritability, low energy and general malaise, and may lead to more serious health situations such as cancer.

CELL PHONES AND EMF

Cell phones emit radio frequency energy, or radio waves, which is a form of electromagnetic radiation. When you put a phone to your ear, it delivers harmful EMFs to your brain, ear, jaws, eyes, teeth, scalp, etc. Most wireless headsets can either concentrate or add to these fields, which may further increase your risk of cancer from these devices.

Scientific data has proven that cell phones are harmful. To protect billion-dollar profits of manufacturers and service providers, this data has been suppressed. Recent clinical and laboratory studies have shown that the EMF radiation emitted from cell phones can cause conditions such as:

Headache	Sleep disruption
Alzheimer's Disease	Brain tumors
Parkinson's Disease	Altered memory function
Concentration deficits	Altered spatial awareness
Mild depression (disruption of melatonin, dopamine, and serotonin levels)	

Suggestions:

- **Use the speakerphone.** This is not practical if you are in a public place. Not all cell phones have speakerphones. The sound is often poor.

- **Keep your phone as far from your body as possible.** The worst place to put a cell phone is next to your head/brain. Any part of the body exposed to radiation over long periods can adversely affect it. Others sitting a few feet away during transmission are also exposed to EMFs.

- **Limit cell phone use, and turn it off if not needed.** The cell phone is constantly searching for signals while it is on. If you must keep it on, keep it in another room.

- **Static-field phone protector diodes.** These can convert harmful EMFs into biologically harmless fields. Radiation protectors can also be used to protect you and your family from a TV, land phones, cell phones, computers, and other EMF emitters.

"We don't know the millionth part of one per cent about anything. We don't know what water is. We don't know what light is. We don't know what gravitation is. We don't know what enables us to keep us on our feet when we stand up. We don't know what electricity is. We don't know what heat is. We don't know anything about magnetism. We have a lot of hypotheses about these things, but that is all. But we don't let our ignorance deprive us of their use!" *Thomas A. Edison*

"If all the electricity were suddenly removed from the human body, it would turn to ash." *Biologic Ionization as Applied to Human Nutrition*

Toxic Chemicals

(from "The ABC's of Toxic Chemicals" by Dr. Joyce Woods)

> Dr. Joyce Woods has worked as a medical/surgical nurse, public health nurse, nurse educator, nursing school administrator, occupational health consultant and holds Bachelor of Nursing, Bachelor of Arts (Specialist), and Master of Education degrees. She has also completed her doctoral degree in the area of "Indoor Air Pollution and... it's effect on your health."

Household chemicals cause all kinds of symptoms from panic attacks, anxiety, and bed wetting to cardiovascular problems. Think of your home as a toxic waste dump. The average home today contains 62 toxic chemicals – more than a turn-of-the-century chemistry lab. Over 72,000 synthetic chemicals have been produced since WWII, and less than 2% of these have been tested for toxicity, mutagenic or carcinogenic properties, or birth defects.

In fact, the majority of chemicals have never been tested for long-term effects. EPA studies found that airborne toxic chemicals in household cleaners are 3 times more likely to cause cancer than outdoor air contaminants and concluded that indoor air was 3 to as much as 70 times more polluted than outdoor air.

The Canada Mortgage and Housing Corporation reports that houses today are so energy efficient that "out gassing" of chemicals from construction materials has no where to go, and so it builds up inside the home. We spend 90% of our time indoors, 65% in our homes. And moms, infants, and the elderly spend as much as 90% of their time in the home.

The National Cancer Association released results of a 15 year study concluding that women who work in the home are at a 54% higher risk of developing cancer than women who work outside the home. Cancer rates have almost doubled since 1960, and cancer is now the number one cause of death in children.

There has been a 26% increase in breast cancer since 1982. Breast cancer is the number one killer of women between the ages of 35 and 54. Most likely culprits are household chemicals such as laundry detergents, cleaners, and pesticides. There has been a call from the U.S./Canadian Commission to ban bleach throughout North America, as bleach has been linked to the rising rates of breast cancer in women, reproductive problems in men, and learning and behavioral problems in children.

Chemicals get into our body through inhalation, ingestion, and absorption. We breathe 10 to 20 thousand liters of air per day, and there are more than 3 million poisonings every year. Household cleaners are the number one cause of poisoning children.

Since 1980, the incidence of asthma has increased by 600%. The Canadian Lung Association and the Asthma Society of Canada identify common household cleaners and cosmetics as triggers.

ADD/ADHD are epidemic in schools today. Behavioral problems have long been linked to exposure to toxic chemicals and molds. The use of Ritalin has skyrocketed since 1990.

Labeling laws do not protect the consumer – they protect big business. The New York Poison Control Center reports that 85% of product warning labels were either inadequate or incorrect for identifying a poison and for first aid instructions. Pesticides only have to include active ingredients on the labels, even though the inert (inactive) ingredients may account for 99%, many of which are also toxic poisons.

Chemical and environmental sensitivities are known to cause all types of headaches. Formaldehyde, phenol, benzene, toluene, and xylene are found in common household cleaners, cosmetics, beverages, fabrics, and cigarette smoke. These chemicals are cancer causing and toxic to the immune system.

Chemicals are attracted to, and stored in, the body's fatty tissues. The brain is a prime destination for these destructive organics because of its high fat content and very rich blood supply. The National Institute of Occupational Safety and Health has found that more than 2,500 chemicals in cosmetics are toxic and can cause tumors throughout the body, reproductive complications, biological mutations, and skin and eye irritations.

Fibromyalgia, chronic fatigue syndrome, arthritis, lupus, multiple sclerosis, circulatory disorders, Alzheimer's disease, Parkinson's disease, irritable bowel syndrome, depression, and hormonal problems are diseases commonly related to chemical exposure.

DEADLY CHEMICAL COMPOUNDS

Pesticides and herbicides may not kill only one target organism but will probably also seriously damage or mutate a whole host of others. These compounds tend to stay on the fruit, vegetable, or plant for extended periods. And toxins from our water, air, food, and buildings only make things worse.

Most pesticides are known carcinogens. Some pose as counterfeit versions of the female hormone estrogen. These xenoestrogens may promote hormone-related cancers by stimulating estrogen receptors in the body.

Animal growth hormones used in livestock are another cause for concern. They do not disappear after an animal is butchered, prepared for market, or cooked. They go to our stomachs and affect our bodies. Nor do antibiotics disappear from the milk of a treated cow. It is estimated that one glass of commercial, non-organic milk purchased from a grocery story may contain the residues of up to 100 different antibiotics!

Beyond the hormones and antibiotics that are injected directly into the animal, many of the meats that we eat come from animals fed with antibiotic-laden feeds. Growth hormones in our food supply are blamed for the abnormally early menses of young girls and for the overabundance of female hormones in young men. (Female hormones are given to milk cows to increase production.)

Hybridized foods are also unhealthy and could cause dangerous symptoms. God says to eat every seed-bearing plant after its own kind. Hybridized seedless watermelons, grapes, or other fruits cannot reproduce, and they may not be the healthy food sources that we think they are. *(from "Toxic Relief", Don Colbert, MD, Lake Mary, FL: Siloam, 2001)*

Smoking has the greatest effect on the liver because of the carbon monoxide – the most harmful thing about smoking. To put it bluntly, in order to help someone who smokes improve body chemistry, they must stop smoking. There is no body chemistry program that can counteract the carbon monoxide affects of smoking. *(from Biologic Ionization as applied to Human Nutrition, Alexander F. Beddoe, DDS, p.36)*

At the first puff, the body does not say, "Oh, how wonderful, how beneficial, how pleasant." Instead, it rebels with coughing, perhaps nausea or other signs that this is a harmful substance. However, by ignoring these warning signals and continuing to smoke, pretty soon these warning sentinels are knocked down, and before long, the whole body is out of balance due to the harmful effects of this substance. A similar process takes place with the misuse of alcohol, salt, sugar, and various mixtures of food and most drugs.

TOXINS IN FOODS

Seafood is loaded with toxic mercury and other poisons. Shellfish can be contaminated with parasites and resistant viruses that may not even be killed by high heat. These creatures are considered scavenger animals, which means they consume foods that may be harmful for you. Fried seafood (shrimp, clams, oysters, lobsters, etc.) has the added issue of trans fat and acrylamide.

It is nice to know that Alaskan red salmon is wild and has been proven through independent lab testing to be free of harmful levels of mercury and other contaminants.

AIR POLLUTION IN THE HOME

Our homes should have a complete change of air 3 or 4 times a day. Leave the windows open on each side of the house for better cross ventilation.

Inert (inactive) ingredients in products are protected by trade secrets and are very dangerous. In the work place, Material Safety Data Sheets must accompany any product used. The work place and the outdoors are considered legally-protected environments, while the air inside of private homes is not.

The ideal level of relative humidity in the home is between 35% and 45%. Anything higher causes mold. When we use humidifiers or dehumidifiers with standing water, we are encouraging the growth of mold.

The ideal temperature in the home is between 68 and 78°F. Anything higher makes chemicals more active. And when we shower, the hot water combined with chlorine in the water can cause major headaches.

Steam from our dryer vents may be extremely toxic because of the chemicals from dryer sheets and the residues from laundry soap and bleach.

Chemicals used to dry clean clothing are very dangerous and can cause cancer. When you bring dry cleaning home, you should hang it outside for at least 3 days. Dry-cleaning chemicals are the same cancer causing chemicals that are found in moth balls. Chemicals found in aerosols are also dangerous and can cause dizziness.

There are roughly 4700 chemicals in tobacco smoke, and volatile chemicals, such as formaldehyde, from carpets and plastics have been found to cause kidney and liver damage.

Some products that contain formaldehyde:

Antiperspirants	Baggies
Mouthwash	Permanent press clothing
Toothpaste	Floor waxes
Tupperware®	Furniture polishes
Wax paper	Coffee
Money	

Formaldehyde can cause allergies, asthma, cancer, and immune system deficiency.

Some products that contain phenols:

Acne medication	Wallpaper
Baking Powder	Mouthwash
Sugar substitutes	TV sets
Computers	

Phenols are absorbed by the lungs and skin and can cause caustic burns, kidney and liver damage, and hyperactivity (besides being possibly fatal).

Lysol also contains phenols – and dioxin, a component of Agent Orange! Lysol is far more dangerous than we thought. Even air fresheners desensitize the nerves in your nose so you cannot smell.

Fungicides used on fruit trees in the Okanagan, BC and in south-western Ontario have been found to be the cause babies in these areas being born with no eyes or very tiny eyes.

When using chlorine, antiseptics, or bleach in industrial areas, you are required to wear impervious protective clothing, hard hats, boots, gloves, apron or coveralls, and chemical goggles or full face shield and use only in well ventilated areas. Such precautions are rarely, if ever, taken in the home.

When using Easy Off, make sure all of your skin is covered, wear protective clothing, do not breath in the fumes, and don't get it on your enamel. (If this product will harm the enamel on your stove, can you imagine what it will do to us.)

Nitrilotriacetic acid (NTA), a substitute for phosphates used in detergents to create suds, was banned from use, but Proctor &

Gamble successfully lobbied to bring back the use of NTA in 1980. More suds mean less clean, however, and more toxic danger. Studies on the suds in toothpaste found these suds to be from laundry detergent, as well.

Eliminating the cause of the environmental illness is more effective (prevention, 80-90% effective compared to treatment, 50-60% effective) and much less expensive than treating the symptom. But our immune system is also very powerful, like a janitorial system, and giving our bodies good nutrition means our body can repair itself and will be able to handle what we face in the world.

Natural Cleaning Alternatives

(Also check out this website: www.nokout.com)

KEEPING THE OVEN CLEAN

To keep an oven clean, use aluminum foil under casseroles, pie pans, and baking dishes. If food boils over, it falls into the foil and not to the oven floor. Wipe down the oven after each use or whenever you wash dishes and wipe the counters.

WINDOW CLEANER

Water alone works very well on most window grime. If you have grease, propane, or natural gas deposits, use a quarter cup or more of vinegar to a gallon of water. Baking soda will remove things that insist on sticking to the window. Mix with water to make a paste, and scrub the area. Rinse with clear water. Or use a nylon scrubber dipped in hot vinegar. If your windows have been neglected and are in really bad shape, use washing soda and water (about a tablespoon per quart of water), and rinse well.

Here is another suggestion that can double as a degreaser and is especially handy in the kitchen. Combine in a spray bottle. Shake to blend.

¼ cup vinegar (distilled, white, 5%)

½ teaspoon liquid soap or detergent

2 cups of water

FLOOR CLEANER

For hard surface floors, use vinegar at the rate of ¼ to ½ cup to a gallon of warm water will clean as well as many commercial cleaners. For the toughest dirt, drip or spray vinegar full strength, then mop it up. Another way to attack dirt is to use a quick squirt of dish detergent or a teaspoon of laundry detergent in a half gallon of water.

SINK, TUB, AND HARD SURFACE CLEANER

Put baking soda into a container with a shaker type of lid, like an empty spice bottle or a salt shaker. Wet the surface, and sprinkle baking soda on it. Scrub, and rinse well. The gentle abrasion of baking soda will make porcelain and stainless steel shine! If you need something to remove stains, add one part hydrogen peroxide mixed with two parts water to the baking soda after sprinkling it on the surface to be cleaned. Measure in teaspoons, not cups.

BATHROOM WALL AND SHOWER TILE CLEANER

Dish detergent, mixed at a 1:1 ratio with warm water, will clean soap scum and light mold from shower tile. It will only take a couple of tablespoons of cheap detergent – that's all you need to cover the walls. Use a scrub brush for the quickest job, and rinse by pouring water over the tile. Wall tile can be cleaned the same way, just use a cloth to rinse instead.

FURNITURE CLEANER AND POLISH

Mix two parts of olive oil and one part white vinegar in a blender to emulsify. Put a little on wood furniture then rub it in. Wipe off the excess. You can substitute lemon juice for vinegar. It smells better, but it's not as frugal.

CLEANING CLOTHS

Make cleaning cloths by cutting old material to size and hemming. Use only absorbent materials – white or colorfast for use with bleach. Wash and reuse. They are more environmentally friendly and easier on your plumbing, flooring, and any other surface.

SOFT SCRUB (for the bathtub, shower, and stainless steel)

In a bowl, stir ½ cup of baking soda and liquid soap or detergent until the consistency reaches that of frosting. Scoop the creamy mixture onto a sponge, wash the surface with it, and rinse. 5 drops antibacterial essential oil such as lavender, tea tree oil, or rosemary is optional.

ALL-PURPOSE CLEANER (super heavy-duty alkaline cleaning)

> ½ teaspoon washing soda
> A dab of liquid soap
> 2 cups hot tap water

Combine the ingredients in a spray bottle, and shake to dissolve the washing soda. Apply and wipe off with a sponge or rag.

Vinegar and Baking Soda

Vinegar is a mildly bleaching, antiseptic, mineral-loaded acid. It neutralizes alkali in soaps and detergents, which makes a good balancing rinse for hair, clothing, and floors. It preserves food against dangerous bacteria, cuts through grease, deodorizes, and disinfects.

Baking soda is a naturally occurring mild abrasive and can be substituted for anything that is abrasive – pot and pan scrubber, sink cleaner, and some recommend using as a toothpaste. (I personally do not recommend scrubbing teeth with baking soda as it can cause sensitivity.)

Naturally alkaline, baking soda is an acid neutralizer. Heartburn goes away when you down a half teaspoon of baking soda mixed into a half glass of water. Test your garden soil for acidity by mixing one cup of soil with two cups water, then stirring in ¼ cup of baking soda. Soil is very acid if it erupts in the container. If it fizzes a little around the edges, it is minimally acidic. Mix it into a litter box, put it in the refrigerator, or spray it (dissolved in water) into the air, and it is an odor neutralizer.

Smothering a grease fire and scrubbing away burned on food are claims made for common salt as well as baking soda, but use a little common sense when trying these ideas.

Vinegar Uses:

(Straight 5% distilled white vinegar can also be sprayed directly onto areas to be cleaned or deodorized. Don't rinse!)

- Fabric softener and static cling reducer - use as you would liquid fabric softener.

- Window cleaner - mix ¼ cup of white vinegar with 2 cups of water. Soak a small sponge or cloth in it, then wring out and store in an airtight container. Use to wipe off spots or smears.

- Air freshener, used with baking soda - use 1 teaspoon baking soda, 1 tablespoon vinegar, and 2 cups of water. After it stops foaming, mix well, and use in a (recycled) spray bottle into the air.

- Chewing gum dissolver - saturate the area with vinegar. If the vinegar is heated, it will work faster.

- Stain remover - for stains caused by grass, coffee, tea, fruits, and berries.

- Corn and callus remover - soak a piece of stale bread (a cloth would probably do as well) in vinegar, and tape it over the callus or corn overnight.

- Age spot fader - Mix equal parts of onion juice and vinegar, and use daily on age spots. It will take a few weeks to work. Just like it's expensive relative from the store

- Hard water deposit remover - For porcelain, chrome, or other hard surface, soak a rag in vinegar, and put it over the area. Leave it overnight. In the morning, the deposits will wipe off. In your steam iron, run vinegar through it instead of water. Hold it a few inches from the surface of your ironing board, and let it steam away. Chunks of deposits will be spit out.

- Mold Fighter - Pour white distilled vinegar into a spray bottle, spray on the moldy area, and let set without rinsing. The smell will dissipate in a few hours. This will, reportedly, kill 82% of mold.

- Deodorizer, Toilet Bowl Cleaner – Vinegar is an acidic cleaning powerhouse. Heinz references studies that say vinegar kills 99% of bacteria, 82% of mold, and 80% of germs.

Baking Soda Uses:

- Soothe bee stings by mixing with water to make a thick paste, then cover the sting area with it.

- Pot scrubber – make it into a paste, and scrub stainless steel, iron, or copper pots and bottoms with it. Do not use on aluminum.

- Antacid – Mix ½ teaspoon in about 4 ounces of water, and drink all at one time. It will neutralizes stomach acid the same way it does other acids.

- Carpet deodorizer – sprinkle on carpet, leave overnight, then vacuum in the morning. Offending odors will be gone.

- Facial scrub – Use a paste, and massage gently into the skin. Rinse with water. (Wipe with vinegar if you want to be sure to remove all traces, then rinse again.)

- Battery acid neutralizer – quickly neutralize spilled battery acid by sprinkling generously with baking soda.

THE BENEFITS OF PEROXIDE VERSUS BLEACH

Bleach was invented in the late 40's. It contains chlorine, which was used to kill troops. Bleach smells bad and is not healthy.

Peroxide was invented during WWI in the 20's. It was used to save and cleanse the wounds of our troops and was used in hospitals as an antiseptic. A bottle of 3% hydrogen peroxide can be purchased for under $1.00.

- Take one capful, and hold in your mouth for 10 minutes daily, then spit it out. Your teeth will be whiter, and it helps to heal canker sores. Use it instead of mouthwash.

- Soak your toothbrushes in a cup of peroxide to keep them free of germs.

- Clean your counters and table tops with peroxide to kill germs and leave a fresh smell. Put a little on your dishrag when you wipe, or spray it on the counters.

- After rinsing off your wooden cutting board, pour peroxide on it to kill salmonella and other bacteria.

- For fungus on toes or feet, spray a 50/50 mixture of peroxide and water every night, and let dry.

- Soak any infections or cuts in 3% peroxide for five to ten minutes, several times a day.

- Fill a spray bottle with a 50/50 mixture of peroxide and water, and keep it in every bathroom to disinfect without harming your septic system.

- Tilt your head back, and spray a 50/50 mixture into your nostrils whenever you have a cold or plugged sinuses. It will bubble and help to kill the bacteria. Hold for a few minutes, and then blow your nose into a tissue.

- If you have a terrible toothache and cannot get to a dentist right away, put a capful of 3% peroxide into your mouth, and hold it for ten minutes several times a day. The pain will lessen greatly.

- For a natural look to your hair, spray the 50/50 solution on your wet hair after a shower, and comb it through. As it gradually lightens, there will be more natural highlights for light brown or dirty blonde hair.

- Put half a bottle of peroxide in your bath to help get rid of boils, fungus, or other skin infections.

- Add a cup of peroxide instead of bleach to a load of whites in your laundry to whiten them. Pour it directly on blood on clothing. Let it sit for a minute, then rub it, and rinse with cold water. Repeat if necessary.
- Clean mirrors. There is no smearing.

Conclusion

"Now the [Bereans] were of more noble character than [the Thessalonians], for they received the message with great eagerness and examined the Scriptures every day to see if what Paul said was true." *Acts 17:11 NIV*

My purpose for writing this book has been to enable you to become an active participant in your own health. I pray you will fulfill your purpose and use your God-given talents as you become free of physical ailments, emotional issues, or spiritual limitation. Let this be a starting point, a challenge, a bridge for you to take the next step. Walk away from disease and sickness into health. Allow me to help you visualize that next step.

Imagine yourself in a garden of flowers and trees, beautiful and sweet smelling. The garden is at its peak, and every type and kind of flower, tree, and vegetation blossoms and yields delightful colors and scents.

But the season must end, and the harsh winter looms nearby. Standing in the midst of those lifeless flowers, your desire is to have that garden come alive and to enjoy the fresh, sweet smells again. But the season drifts slowly by, never to return to the beauty it once boasted.

As you walk away from that garden of wilted, deteriorated, and sun-scorched flowers, you see a long, long, wooden bridge that is shaky and insecure. Below the bridge is a swift turbulence of deep, troubled waters. You look down, and you become anxious and fearful.

You have choices. You have been told that on the other side of the bridge is a never-ending garden of fresh blossoms, colorful vegetables and fruits, and a new day. The bridge is shaky and weak, but the old garden is finished, dead, and lifeless. You struggle with questions and fear.

As you decide to push forward, you say a prayer and cautiously step onto the bridge with one final glance backwards. Each step is frightening and scary, and it seems like such a long journey. Finally you can see the garden and everything you wanted is ahead. You step onto the terrain with a sigh and a feeling of relief. You take a deep breath, and it overwhelms you – the strong fragrance of victory!

Envision yourself, well and healthy, doing those things that the Lord has called upon you to do. Feeling good, the task before you is now a reality. Your body, emotions, and spirit line up with faith, courage, and hope. You are living in victory!

May God Richly Bless You

Kathy Stricker

Recommended Reading

BOOKS

"Why Christians Get Sick" by Dr. George H. Malkmus

"Eat Right For Your Type" by Dr. Peter J. D'Adamo

"A Cancer Battle Plan" by Anne E. Frahm.

"Discovering Wholeness" by Dr. Cheryl Townsley

"What Would Jesus Eat?" Don Colbert, MD

"Heinerman's Encyclopedia of Healing Juices" by John Heinerman

"Herbal Teas" by Kathleen Brown

"Planetary Herbology" by Michael Tierra

"The ABC Herbal" by Steven H. Horne

"The ProVita! Plan" by Jack Tips

"Colon Health" by Dr. Norman W. Walker

"Diet & Nutrition: A Holistic Approach" by Rudolph Ballentine

"Natural Health Remedies" by Janet Maccaro

"Worst Pills, Best Pills" by Sidney M. Wolfe, Larry D. Sasich, and Rose-Ellen Hope

"The Complete Encyclopedia of Natural Healing" by Gary Null

"Prescription for Nutritional Healing" by James F. Balch and Phyllis A. Balch

"Kid Smart!" by Cheryl Townsley

"Eating for A's" by Alexander Schauss, Barbara Friedlander Meyer, and Arnold Meyer

"The Roots of Health" by L. Carl Robinson

"Earthly Bodies & Heavenly Hair" by Dina Falconi

"Essential Oils Desk Reference", Essential Science Publishing

"Heinerman's New Encyclopedia of Fruits & Vegetables" by John Heinerman

WEB SITES

www.herbsbymerlin.com

www.mercola.com

www.naturessunshine.com (Please enter sponsor code 877221.)

www.fromnaturewithlove.com

www.hmbeautyrecipes.homestead.com

www.ourhealthcoop.com

www.debralynndadd.com

www.pureherbs.com

www.safecosmetics.org

www.healthline.cc

www.seventhgeneration.com

www.mountainroseherbs.com

www.youngliving.com (Please enter sponsor code 222750.)

www.precisionherbs.com

Index

Index

"Many are trying to have health without the God of life and health. Sort of like trying to defy the law of gravity without a parachute. There is no neutral ground. If you are not actively choosing God, your life will be directed much like a computer. That is, it will default from God's program to programs of disease, unhappiness, nonfulfillment, etc., which operate in the false beliefs and misunderstandings of your mind. In effect, that is just like choosing to pull the plug on your own power supply. The state of things change. Instead of life without end, there is an end to life. Separation from God – truth – is the separation from the source of life. If we separate from the source of life we begin our process toward losing life. Choosing to separate from God and going alone is to cut yourself off, thus beginning the process of suffocation."

– Biological Ionization As Applied To Human Nutrition, Dr. A.F. Beddoe

31181158R10131

Made in the USA
Middletown, DE
21 April 2016